The
Shrinkology
Solution

Publishing Director **Sarah Lavelle**
Commissioning Editor **Susannah Otter**
Designer **Jim Smith**
Cover Design **David Eldridge**
Production Director **Vincent Smith**
Production Controller **Tom Moore**

Published in 2018 by Quadrille,
an imprint of Hardie Grant Publishing

Quadrille
52–54 Southwark Street
London SE1 1UN
quadrille.com

Cataloguing in Publication Data: a catalogue record
for this book is available from the British Library.

Text © Dr Meg Arroll and Louise Atkinson 2018
Design © Quadrille 2018

ISBN 978 1 78713 184 2

Printed in Italy

The information contained in this book is for educational purposes only.
It is the result of the study and experience of the authors. Whilst the information
and advice offered are believed to be true and accurate at the time of going to press,
neither the authors nor the publisher can accept any legal responsibility or liability
for any errors or omissions that may have been made of for any adverse effects which
may occur as a result of following the recommendations given herein. Always consult
a qualified medical practitioner if you have any concerns regarding your health.

The Shrinkology Solution

Discover your eating type,
lose weight and
keep it off – for life

DR MEG ARROLL AND LOUISE ATKINSON

quadrille

Contents

Preface

When we were introduced to each other at a pre-Christmas party at the end of 2016, we quickly established a mutual interest in the psychology of dieting. Louise had long harboured a fantasy to write *the* diet book to end all diet books: the definitive, easy and effective, no hunger or hardship route to effortless slenderness. But having read and written about diets for decades, and having seen her own weight yo-yo as she diligently tried them all, she had become convinced there was no such thing as **the** perfect diet plan.

Something became clear. The issue rarely lies with the diet – it lies with the dieter.

Together, we talked about the extent to which the success of any weight-loss programme must inevitably depend on the complicated mix of factors which combine to create an individual's pattern of eating behaviour, personality and circumstance.

It was like a serendipitous meeting of minds – Meg had a fascinatingly insightful, robust and research-based answer to every question Louise fired at her. It became clear that any attempts at weight loss might work in the short term (as so many diets will) but are destined to fail unless you have your head in the right place, you address any possible 'issues' that might subconsciously be affecting your eating behaviour, you pick a diet plan that fits your personality, lifestyle and circumstances and, crucially, which works so seamlessly as part of your life that you are able to incorporate elements into your eating long term and maintain a happy, healthy weight forever.

And so Shrinkology was born as an insightful way to understand what we called 'the psychology of slim'. If you want to shrink (lose weight, tighten up, get healthy) you need to start thinking like a 'shrink'.

While any diet might restrict your calorie intake, it will rarely change your relationship with food or deal with the underlying psychological reasons that entice you to overeat, or break your resolve. We are convinced that Shrinkology is the key to ensuring you pick the right diet, stick at it more effectively, lose weight and actually keep it off. It is the missing extra layer in the dieting process, the expert and essential filter between 'I really want to lose weight' and 'this is the diet for me'.

Whether you have always struggled with your weight or you are concerned about the eating habits of a partner, child, parent or friend, Shrinkology will empower you with psychological insight.

We are convinced that the Shrinkology solution also adds an important new voice to the obesity debate, and we hope it will help medics understand the complex psychological processes that contribute to the escalating obesity problem, helping to support patients on their weight-loss journey.

Thirty million Brits attempt to lose weight every year. The vast majority fail – less than five per cent of those who go on a diet will keep the weight off. The rest of us want to know why and what we can do about it.

We believe Shrinkology holds the key.

How to use this book

We have put blood, sweat and tears into every word on every page of this book, so, not surprisingly, we want you to read it all. You will certainly get the most from the Shrinkology message if you start at the beginning and read steadily through to the end.

Between us, we know a bit about psychology and the slimming mentality, and so we know that there's a pretty strong chance you will want to find your very own quick-fix Shrinkology solution. By all means take the quiz (see page 71) to find which of the 6 Shrinkology types applies to you, gaining insight into the deep-seated principles that subconsciously guide your behaviour when it comes to food, then turn straight to your type chapter. There you'll find specifically tailored behavioural and dietary advice to suit the nuances of your eating personality, plus tailored exercise and activity recommendations to enhance your personalised plan.

This will mean that you'll be able to hit the ground running straight away – but you do risk missing out on the fundamentals which underpin everything you'll learn. When you have a quiet moment we would urge you to got through the rest of the book.

Part 1 lays out the Shrinkology Scenario and the shocking plethora of factors conspiring to encourage us all to gain weight. There is reassurance in the research, which shows how resilient you can be – given the right guidance – in the face of this onslaught.

Part 2 teaches you how to become your own Shrinkologist, with details on how to create a food/mood diary (see page 60) as a way to gain insight into your own eating behaviours. Once you have realised the inextricable link between the food you eat and your mood, take the quiz (see page 71) to discover your type and spend a little time cherry picking from the Shrinkology Fundamentals chapter, which will provide a properly strong foundation to what we confidently hope will be your serious, long-term weight-loss journey.

Part 3 dedicates one chapter to each Shrinkology type. Although you are most likely to fall firmly into one of the six categories, there will be aspects of your lifestyle and personality that involve influences from the others. It is certainly worth reading through the chapters for Shrinkology types other than your own. You will find great hacks and tips that will work for you – and fantastic snippets of advice you might want to pass on to others.

Part 4 explains how your Shrinkology type can evolve and change as you go through life.

If you enjoy this book and find it as useful as we hope you will, please spread the word. Tell everyone you can about your Shrinkology success and urge the important people in your life to follow their own Shrinkology journey. Check out our website – **www.shrinkology.co.uk** – for more insight and advice, constantly updated expert verdicts and type-specific recommendations on the latest popular diet plans as they appear. Please follow us on Twitter @shrinksolution and Instagram @shrinkologysolution and become part of the happy, healthy Shrinktastic community worldwide.

Time to think 'shrink'

Weightloss is a totally personal journey. Whether you want to drop a few pounds so your summer swimsuit still flatters, or you are on doctor's orders to drastically change your body shape; whether you are confounded by the slow creep of a steadily expanding waistline or the fact that your favourite fall-back diet plan is now suddenly failing you; whether you're terrified of feeling hungry or missing out on the delicious food you love – everyone is different.

Whatever your motivation, your health should be key. It is not healthy to be overweight, but neither is it healthy to desperately searching for some impossibly skinny ideal. Shrinkology is not about achieving the perfect size, whatever that is for you, sporting a washboard stomach or catwalk emaciation. It's not even about being in uncommonly great shape for a man or woman of your age.

A far, far better goal should be to find, reach and maintain a healthy weight for *you*.

There's every chance if you're reading this that you're not completely happy with your body shape or size, and that diets for you may have seen mixed success over the years.

If being slimmer is a positive healthy goal which will ultimately benefit both your mental and physical health then the key to your future success and to effective and long-term shrinkage could lie in learning to think like a diet 'shrink'.

Why it's not just a question of eating less and moving more

All the evidence suggests that many diets DO work[1] – for a while. Weight loss is all about creating a calorie deficit, and whether you're cutting out carbohydrates, skipping meals or feverishly logging fat grams, your diet plan of choice will have been designed to create a situation where you eat less energy than you expend. But even the best slimming regimes have an appallingly low long-term success rate. No matter how convinced we are that the latest 'miracle' weight-loss plan is going to work, how efficiently we stock the kitchen with kale or protein powder, matcha or crispbreads, even the strongest willpower can only sustain us for so long. In the end, the inevitable weeks of hunger and social isolation bite hard. We slip up, stumble and somehow find ourselves face first in a bowl of trifle.

What we fail to fully appreciate is the fact that it is very rarely poor willpower or self-control, sloth or gluttony causing those diets to fail. It is much more likely to be deep-seated emotional and behavioural traits which conspire to lead you to subconsciously sabotage your own best-laid plans. In short, you probably picked the wrong diet for your personality type.

Despite all the hype regularly trotted out by the media, there's no such thing as the perfect diet and no one-size-fits-all, 100% effective weight-loss regime. Advances in nutritional science mean the healthy eating messages keep changing (low-fat/high-fat, carbs are good/carbs are bad, salt is bad/salt is good) and we have never been more confused and bewildered. Add to this the popularity of the beautiful, young 'clean eating' brigade which has left a generation of 'orthorexics' (see page 141) who shun whole food groups but line the pockets of the food manufacturers happily stocking up the 'free from' aisles.

It is quite clear that weight management is not one single problem that can be fixed by one holy grail 'perfect diet' solution. Anyone who has ever dieted knows it's not that simple.

Fundamental to the success of any weight-management plan but rarely discussed in the diet world is the fact that personality and circumstance, as well as emotional and behavioural characteristics, need to be factored into the mix. That's where the Shrinkology Solution comes in. In an era of increasing credence on personalised medicine, Shrinkology offers the first expertly researched and extremely readable guide to creating a bespoke and truly personalised long-term diet for life.

Shrinkology not only provides the rationale behind using your mind to change your body, crucially, it shows you how. This book will help you harness the power of psychology and will encourage you to become your own insightful diet 'shrink'. You will discover a unique insight into your own deeply entrenched attitudes to food, helping you select the best diet plan most likely to succeed long term. Shrinkology then supports your weight-loss journey with clever individually targeted tips, tricks and life skills to support you in overcoming any emotional or situational triggers, end the scourge of yo-yo dieting and achieve successful physical 'shrinkage' that might have eluded you so far.

Learning to become 'Shrinktastic' is about discovering your own triggers, incentives and rewards; it is about guiding you to a happy place where you are content with your body, confident that it is as healthy as it can be – regardless of the size label on the back of your jeans. Using the research and principles of psychology, Shrinkology establishes six distinct overeating categories: The Gourmet (who lives to entertain and indulge); The Magpie (flitting from one sparkly new diet plan to another); The Rebel (who throws everything at a diet, only to abandon it spectacularly at the first glitch); The Scrambler (forever nibbling, grazing, snacking on the hoof); The Soother (who finds comfort and solace in food), and The Traditional (adhering to deeply established dietary conventions).

Knowing your type gives you a unique insight into the deep-seated principles which subconsciously guide your behaviour when it comes to food – because you are the best judge of your own eating behaviours and you are the only one who can remedy them. For a diet to work long term it has to include foods you like, fit the lifestyle you lead and suit your type, or you just won't be able to stick at it.

Dr. Caroline Apovian, who is the highly acclaimed director of the nutrition and weight management centre at Boston Medical Centre in the US, has wisely said most people can lose weight but keeping it off is the key. Finding something that works, she says, has always been a case of trial and error. We are convinced that Shrinkology will funnel you closer to finding the right solution as it effectively restricts that trial and hugely constricts your potential for error.

This book will not be adding to the quagmire of confusion by inventing a new method of food restriction, and calling it 'miraculous' or 'life-changing'. This is not a quick-fix 'lose a stone in a month' diet book, but a robust, expertly researched and extremely readable guide to creating a bespoke long-term diet solution. *The Shrinkology Solution* will provide you with a truly personalised, expert guide to picking the perfect diet plan with personality-focused tips and tricks to end the scourge of yo-yo dieting and ensure you find your happy, healthy weight and stay there effortlessly, forever.

Part One
The Shrinkology Scenario

In this section, we've built a comprehensive picture of the many emotional, behavioural, physical and environmental factors conspiring to make dieting difficult. There are a huge amount of influences on the way you eat, many of which operate beneath the radar of your consciousness. With such strong forces conspiring to encourage us to eat more than we physically need, it is quite surprising any of us are able to successfully maintain a healthy, happy weight. Whether these forces are internally generated (Chapter 1) or externally applied (Chapter 2) one thing is certain: they have very real physical consequences. Becoming aware of these sometimes very subtle influences, and recognising the ones that particularly affect you, marks the first and most important step to creating your own personalised Shrinkology solution.

Chapter 1
Why is Dieting so Damned Difficult?

Dieting is tough and if you've been struggling to achieve and maintain a happy healthy body shape it's probably not your fault. So many of our disordered eating patterns are the symptom, rather than the cause, of underlying habits formed in childhood, our attempts to fit in socially, the tricks our body plays to ensure we survive and thrive, reactions to trauma and the subtle ways we battle to cope with all-pervading, modern 24/7 stress.

Your metabolism could be slowing down

Your metabolism is the amount of energy your body burns just to stay alive. Everyone's metabolic rate is subtly different – some burn hot, others burn cold – and the amount of fuel you need to feed that fire will depend on genetics, gender, height, weight and muscle mass, and age. Too much fuel, and you'll be likely to gain weight. In fact, most cases of stubborn middle-aged spread can be blamed on the fact that we continue to eat roughly what we normally eat when our metabolism is dropping roughly one to two percent per decade. After the age of 30 your metabolism will drop by as much as five percent per decade and from the age of 40 that decline will accelerate further.

This drop is perfectly natural as every cell in our body starts to slow down, but it means you'll burn 100 fewer calories per day at the age of 35 than you did at 25, and 200 fewer at 45. This could be enough to trigger an annual weight gain of 3.5–5.5kg (8–12lb).

If you have become increasingly sedentary with age, that lack of activity is only going to slow your metabolism further and make things worse.

When it comes to creating the calorie deficit that will help you lose weight, it is far, far more effective to restrict the calories going in, than rely on burning up enough energy at the gym to deal with your pizza habit. For health, as well as weight loss, the adage 'you can't outrun a bad diet' holds true. But exercise *is* extremely important in the quest to achieve a healthy body, and if you, like so many people today, live a completely sedentary life, you are very likely to find weight loss difficult.

A quarter of adults exercise less than 30 minutes *a week* – not a day, a week.[2] We don't even move around much at home. We have cars to go even short distances, our jobs are rarely physical, and many hobbies and fun activities are static, so exercise is something that generally has to be factored in, and in our ever busy lives, this can be tough.

A sedentary life is extremely unhealthy. In fact, studies show it is even worse for you, in terms of life expectancy, than smoking. And it will certainly be difficult to slow that metabolic decline and maintain a healthy weight without adding bit of activity in the mix.

It could be your hormones

When it comes to weight fluctuations, hormones have a lot to answer for, particularly for women. As any woman over the age of 50 will tell you, menopause can make weight maintenance tricky. Around 90 per cent of menopausal women find they gain up to a stone in weight very gradually during their peri-menopausal years (which can start in the late 30s) as a result of the imbalance of the sex hormones: oestrogen, progesterone and testosterone. Although menopause is most often associated with a drop off in oestrogen, it is more likely to be falling levels of progesterone and testosterone which actually allow oestrogen to become dominant (albeit at a much lower level than before). This makes the body better at storing fat, and inhibits its ability to use fat stores effectively for energy.

In younger women, a condition called Polycystic Ovary Syndrome can cause unwanted and stubborn fat to appear around the middle. Most of the symptoms are triggered by too much testosterone and other male hormones. Sufferers very often also have insulin resistance, which can trigger stubborn weight gain.

It could be your medication

Many drugs are linked to weight gain, including anti-depressants, prescriptions for migraine, diabetes, high blood pressure and the contraceptive pill, but the same medication might push one person's weight up and cause another person's weight to fall. If you are convinced that your weight has increased only since you've been taking medication, check the side-effect profile. If 'possible weight gain' is listed, talk to your GP about trying a suitable alternative.

You could have inherited a 'fat gene'

There is no doubt that a tendency to gain weight runs in families, and although argument rages over the relative influence of nurture over nature (if you've been brought up on pizza, burgers and a fully-stocked 'treats' cupboard, the odds are likely to be stacked against you), many studies have sought to identify specific genes linked to weight gain.

Experts agree that there is a strong genetic component to being overweight, and studies show certain genes can make appetite easier to control. An estimated one in six people has a genetic make-up that is vulnerable to weight gain and as a result weighs an average of 3kg (7lb) more than those who don't, with around 15 per cent more body fat.

One Scottish research team, led by Dr Nik Morton of Edinburgh University, has identified a gene which encourages fat storage, specifically the genes in fat tissue which determine the breakdown or putting down of fat, regardless of diet.

However, confusingly, having these so-called 'fat genes' doesn't necessarily mean you'll struggle to maintain a healthy weight. Lifestyle clearly plays a very important role. Children tend to eat what their parents eat,[3] so if you grew up in a home where snacks and treats were readily available, these will be the types of foods you are also likely to choose. Studies show the eating habits we form as children trickle through adolescence,[4] then into adulthood.[5] This could be due to exposure, because it's hard to develop a taste for healthy foods you've never had the opportunity to try, and the more times a child tastes a new food, the greater the chance of them liking it.[6,7] This is why eating behaviours from childhood can persist and being overweight can run in families. Our brains are hard-wired to use as few resources as possible on everyday decisions like eating so they can concentrate on the bigger issues, such as complex work tasks and social interactions. As a result, we might find ourselves eating on autopilot (see Eating on Autopilot on page 257) and following possibly unhealthy eating patterns from childhood without even realising.

You've yo-yo dieted for years

If you've ever stuck rigidly to a diet, managed to lose weight but then piled the pounds back on, the chances are you're not lazy, greedy or woefully lacking in willpower – it's just that your body is doing what it has evolved to do: fighting back against the perils of potential imminent starvation. In an ideal world your body will defend its healthy weight range with a natural process of subconscious weight regulation that gently nudges hunger and activity levels, so you eat or exercise no more or less than your body needs to maintain this self-defined 'brain weight'. As every inveterate dieter knows, dropping too low might thrillingly squeeze you into your skinny jeans, but it will be fiendishly difficult to maintain. There's every chance your weight will plateau as you meet powerful resistance in the form of cravings for quick-fix calories and energy-conserving listlessness to keep you at this brain weight. You'd think these natural 'starvation!' alerts would only kick in once your ribs started showing, or a thigh gap appeared, but infuriatingly, everyone's brain weight is different.

If you've gained pounds over the years, with successive diets resulting in a gradually expanding waistline, experts believe your brain weight is very likely to have settled at a level far higher than the 'fighting weight' you might so long to return to. This means your brain could regard a drop even to the point of last year's lowest level as threateningly low, and strongly resist your attempts to get there.

The reason is partly evolutionary, because for early man one of the biggest threats to survival was starvation. In times of famine, it made sense to enhance appetite, seek out food, conserve energy (the metabolism slows) and lay down more fat to mitigate the harmful effects of starvation.

Dieting also flicks psychological switches making 'banned' or restricted foods seem super-appealing. Any seasoned dieter will know that the act of cutting back foods is the best possible way to increase your preoccupation with food. There are plenty of studies which show that trying *not* to think about something is one of the best ways to force you to think about it. In fact, when we diet, preoccupation with all types of foods increases, not just the prohibited ones.[8] When researchers ask people to stop eating chocolate, they develop cravings for it and find it harder to concentrate, as the brain focuses on and seeks out what it has been denied.[9] You don't need us to tell you that chocolate, once limited, becomes a much more desirable thing.

Another reason why dieting can be so difficult is what psychologists call 'restraint theory', which explains why we end up overeating specifically when we try not to eat.[10] If you are subconsciously using certain foods as a crutch to help you deal with emotions, stress or boredom, you can very easily come unstuck when you try to remove that food without replacing the food crutch. That's where our Shrinkology hacks come in (see Part 3).

Your hunger signalling could be out of kilter

If you've been really good at dieting in the past, particularly if you've been a fan of fasting diets, there's every chance you've become super efficient at ignoring your body's hunger signals. But this success has a hidden diet flaw: it could mean that when you do eat your body is driven by hunger (and a natural urge to ensure you stock up in times of famine like this) and then it completely overrides the fullness signals when you do sit down to eat, making overeating more likely. It means many habitual dieters end up eating to order, or with complete abandon, because their hunger signalling is hazy and they have no idea whether they are truly hungry or have eaten enough.

If you have steely determination, you can summon all your powers of self-control to get you through the 'fasting' phase of an intermittent fasting programme, or the tough 'cleansing' phase of a detox plan. But stay on the plan too long and it is easy to come unstuck.

This is because the physiology of hunger is still playing away under the surface (and out of your control), but stress and boredom can become layered on top. If you don't search out support to deal with these everyday occurrences – through Shrinkology hacks – it can all come tumbling down.

There is another issue at play here, whether you are a dieter or not. An eminent US medic, Robert Lustig, Professor of Clinical Paediatrics at the University of California, has devised a compelling scientific theory. He believes that anyone who eats too many sugary foods can develop a natural resistance to the hormone leptin, which tells you when to stop eating. Normally, signals from your rapidly filling stomach trigger the release of leptin which tells your brain to send out instructions to put down the knife and fork and push your plate away. But, Lustig says, if you eat a lot of sugar and refined carbohydrates (which your body thinks of as sugar) your insulin levels are likely to be permanently elevated (all part of your body's attempts to move sugar out of your blood) and this affects the leptin signalling process.

For many years scientists thought obesity could be caused by a shortage of leptin – thinking that due to inadequate levels of leptin, overweight people simply never received the message that they were full, and therefore were continually eating far more than they needed. But more recent studies have shown the bigger you are, the more leptin you often have. The problem, according to Professor Lustig, is that many of us become 'leptin resistant' as a direct result of overeating.[11][12]

His theory states that the more you overeat, the more inured you become to leptin and the more food you need to eat to trigger it. This means the cells in the brain which should register leptin (the leptin receptors) become numb and no longer 'read' the signals saying the body is full, but instead assume it is starving – no matter how much food you continue to eat.

In panic, the brain pumps out instructions to increase energy storage (by instigating powerful cravings for high-fat, high-sugar foods because these are the easiest and most immediate forms of energy) and conserve energy usage (by dampening any urge to get up off the sofa and go for a run).

These cravings are made even more intense – and impossible to resist – because leptin is supposed to dampen the feeling of pleasure and enjoyment you get from food. If you are leptin resistant, food never stops tasting delicious, no matter how much of it you eat.

Thankfully, Professor Lustig has shown that by cutting down on sugar in the diet it is possible to improve 'leptin signalling' (the brain's ability to read leptin), stop cravings, put the brakes on food consumption and trigger weight loss.

Your gut bacteria could be imbalanced and unhappy

The study of gut bacteria is growing fast and scientists are beginning to understand the important role played by the trillions of microbes in your gut. This, your microbiome, is a completely individual soup of helpful and less helpful bacteria. It is not only essential to how you digest food, but it can actually provide vital enzymes and vitamins and, it is thought, help control just how many calories you absorb from your food.

The microbes in your gut have a number of functions, but one of the things they do is decide how much energy your body extracts from the food you eat (which can lead to weight gain if you eat the wrong foods). They also control hunger signals, help decide which foods you crave, and help to determine how much your blood sugar goes up and down in response to a meal.

For instance, it is possible that your gut bacteria have a hand in making you choose a doughnut rather than a stick of celery. This is because there are millions of neurons in your gut which communicate with the brain via a very busy 'telephone line' called the vagus nerve, which travels from gut to brain and back again. There's now evidence that your microbes can hack into this system and 'talk' directly to your brain.

Why would your microbes want to sabotage your healthy eating intentions like this? Well, some microbes need sugar to survive, others need fat, and in a bid for self-preservation, they each try to get more of what they need. The more sugar you feed the sugar-eaters, the more they'll shout for it.

Research shows that having a wide range of different species in your gut normally means you are slimmer and healthier. Having a more limited microbiome is associated with being overweight and sickly.[13] In a healthy diverse microbiome all those tiny creatures are clamouring to be heard and, like a gang of children all shouting at once, can cancel out each other's demands and are actually easier for the brain to ignore. If the sugar-lovers' voice is just as loud as that of the fat-lovers, neither gets heard clearly. The problem comes when one group – say, the ones who thrive on junk food – start to dominate. As a gang, these bad guys will now be much noisier and more influential, and by producing chemical signals, generate cravings for junk food that you will find hard to resist.

A healthy microbiome gets increasingly important as we get older as the wear and tear on the gut lining makes it ever more important to look after the gut bacteria in there working on our behalf. The gut is where you absorb nutrients, and you are not what you eat – you are what you absorb. See page 104 for tips on nourishing your microbiome.

Many factors can alter your microbiome, encouraging unhealthy microbes to flourish and increasing your chance of weight gain:

- Poor diet – processed foods are packed with chemicals and preservatives that healthy gut bacteria hate, and lack the fibre they love. It takes just one day of poor eating to change the composition of your microbiome.[14]
- Artificial sweeteners – studies have shown[15] sweeteners can upset and alter your microbiome balance.
- Painkillers – non-steroidal anti-inflammatory drugs (NSAID) such as aspirin and ibuprofen could be playing havoc with your gut bacteria.[16]
- Antibiotics – these disrupt your gut bacteria which can take months to return to normal.[17]
- Excessive drinking – this puts pressure on the liver, which disturbs gut bacteria balance.[18]
- Stress – our microbiome has a role in how we feel,[19] and stress can disturb gut bacteria balance.[20] (A healthy and diverse microbiome can help you cope with stress.)

You find some foods comforting

A need for comfort can drive what we chose to eat. As children, food is often provided as a source of comfort, even when we're not hungry (the biscuit to stem the tears when we fall over, the sweetie tin at Granny's house) and throughout our lives we will find ourselves in situations where food is clearly associated with love, comfort and security. This helps explain why attempts to restrict it through diets can be so difficult.

For instance, the careful planning and preparation of a meal is so often viewed as an expression of love. The ability to provide the gift of food can be very important in terms of identity.[21] Children often tend to associate this caregiving with the food provided. That's a good thing, right? But sometimes, in some people, feelings of comfort and security can become indistinguishable from food and eating.

From weddings to funerals, many of us see food as either a pacifier or a necessary part of our experience. Either way, in our culture, we often associate happiness with eating. Romantic relationships are often punctuated by going out for a meal, the candlelit dinner for two which can be viewed as part of dating/courtship and food, especially rich, decadent food, can be closely entwined with the pleasure of sexual relationships.

On top of this, our brain finds certain food just plain comforting. Some (usually unhealthy) food can have a drug-like impact on the reward systems of the brain.[22] That's because the brain is hard-wired for survival, so any behaviour that increases our chances of survival is likely to trigger a reward or pleasure system, instigating the release of a brain chemical called dopamine. Dopamine makes us feel good, so anything that triggers its release will feel rewarding to us, and we will – almost unconsciously – feel compelled to repeat the behaviour to get that pleasurable feeling again. It is not that different to drug addiction.[23]

However, it is possible to have 'too much of a good thing' and problems can occur when the brain senses that too much dopamine has been released. It will helpfully surge into action, either eliminating dopamine receptors or sending out instructions to reduce the production of dopamine. This might be good for the brain because neurochemical balance is regained, but it means you'll need more of that rewarding substance (whether it is a drug or a doughnut) to get the same dopamine hit. And if you don't get that hit, you might find yourself experiencing a range of unpleasant feelings – which is effectively dopamine withdrawal.

Rewards (whether that's positive feedback or the buzz from a chocolate biscuit) and punishments (including negative feedback or the feelings of withdrawal when the packet of biscuits is empty) are powerful drivers of behaviour.

This is why the taste and the chemical impact of a big bowl of sticky toffee pudding can provide an intense and immediate pleasurable reward which can be significant enough to the brain to outweigh long-term, nagging negative 'feedback' such as 'it's unhealthy and it's going to make me put on weight.'

This effect can be magnified if you've been brought up to associate 'treat foods' with reward. It might be a completely understandable (and usually highly effective) parenting strategy, but the danger is it can put vegetables in the 'chore' category that might just earn an ice-cream reward.[24]

This practice dramatically increases the desirability of the 'reward' food, because it strengthens the neural connections between food and feeling good (it doesn't just taste great, but I get parental approval too!). This association can become so deeply entrenched as we go through life that as adults we unthinkingly 'treat' ourselves with high-sugar and carbohydrate-laden foods.

Using food as the reward for 'being good' can backfire too because it gives the primary message that these reward foods have greatest value. This can so easily spill over to adulthood – who hasn't rewarded themselves with a fancy cupcake or big glass of wine for finishing a tedious report, getting the kids to sleep (finally!) or enduring the in-laws?

Studies show that school systems whereby children collect tokens (which can later be exchanged for prizes) or cash in return for healthy food choices *do* lead to an improvement in healthy eating patterns, but sadly these changes rarely last.[25] The greatest increase in healthy food choices comes when children are given cash rewards on the same day.[26] This implies that an effective reward for swapping out unhealthy food items should be immediate and to work best, it should somehow also trigger the reward centre of the brain.

It might be worth taking a long hard look at the rewards you derive from your close friendships too. Studies show we can be prone to 'weight contagion', whereby attitude to food, weight and dieting is influenced by the people around us. Perhaps your best friend is a 'feeder' or you have established ingrained habits where you always drink Prosecco/beer or eat chocolate/kebabs together. That friendship could be hindering your diet success. One large, long-term U.S. study found that if a man has a male friend who becomes fat, his risk of becoming overweight is doubled.

Did something happen when you were a child?

But it is not just our physiology that may contribute to how we eat – or why it can be so hard to maintain a healthy weight. Things that happen in our lives have a powerful influence on how we feel and behave, sometimes leading to yo-yo dieting and a tricky relation- ship with food. This is because the mind and body are not separate entities, they are part of the same overall system that is 'you'. Our physiological make-up can make us feel hungry or more inclined to turn to food to balance hormone production but our experiences and emotions can have a major impact on how we perceive food and how tempting it appears to us.

Trauma in early life – whether this is 'Big T'-type trauma such as abuse, maltreatment or war, or 'little t' trauma like unresponsive or overly harsh parenting – can have long-lasting adverse effects which can impact the way we eat. We learn about human relation- ships and concepts such as trust, security and the confidence to explore the world from our mothers, fathers, grandparents and other adults when we are children, so childhood influences can be very important. It can certainly help explain common patterns of comfort eating.

Studies have shown that parenting that could be described as distant and disengaged, inconsistent, disorganised or erratic can lead to low self-esteem and body dissatisfaction in the child.[27] In some cases this can lead you to turn to food as a way of coping with difficult feelings of low self-esteem or insecurity. These patterns can continue into adulthood and become so ingrained that it's difficult to disentangle where feelings start and food stops.[28] You might not even know this applies to you, but if you have had what psychologists call 'insecure attachment', then studies show you could be more likely to be influenced by media ideals of body image (see Chapter 2), which can lead to body dissatisfaction.[29]

A stressful childhood could also trigger over-activation of finely balanced stress systems, which can go on to affect the hormones that regulate eating and feeling full.[30] This could trigger a seeming inability to control eating which, in itself, can increase stress levels, creating a vicious loop and uncontrolled weight gain.

Sometimes, personality differences between parent and child can impact later eating behaviours in the child. For instance, if you experience and express emotion differently from your parents, this can skew future relationships with food. An extroverted parent or caregiver, for example, might, with the best intentions in the world, encourage a shy child to be more outgoing, perhaps insisting they go to parties and playgroups when deep down the child needs much more reassurance and support. You couldn't possibly call this poor parenting[31], but a strong disparity in temperament, amongst a range of possible situations in early life, could lead to a heightened propensity to quite literally feed your emotions, specifically with high-calorie treat food in later life.[32]

It seems if you are the sort who struggles to identify, regulate and express emotions, you could find it more difficult to tolerate your own feelings – and food can become an effective way to dampen these strong feelings. It is the classic comfort eating scenario which sees you diving head first into a tub of ice cream when you're feeling grumpy, or seeking to cheer yourself up with chocolate when you're sad.

If there are any unresolved issues lurking deep down in your consciousness that you might not really want to face, you could find that any small trigger brings out the pain. Sometimes it can feel as if the best way to avoid facing those demons is to stuff them back down with food. Refined sugar or starchy foods, which are bulky and will do the job quickly and easily, will be the first to grab because they can offer comfort (in the form of the pleasure chemical dopamine) at the same time.

Under-valuing ourselves can also contribute to unhealthy food choices.[33] We may not feel we are truly worth taking care of, even if we spend a great deal of time and energy looking after the emotional and practical needs of others. Engaging in thought patterns such as 'it doesn't matter if I eat this as I'm rubbish anyway', followed by overeating and then self-recrimination can form a cycle of distress-overeating-distress. But it is possible to break free of this cycle. Overcoming negative thought patterns can make a big difference to our emotional regulation in the here and right now, setting us free from past influences.

You could be stressed

Stress is an insidious factor in creeping weight gain and if you live a stressful life, you could find maintaining a happy healthy weight difficult. That's because when the body is tense it triggers an over-production of the stress hormones adrenaline and cortisol, both of which can trick the body into thinking it needs to eat. Not only that, stress reduces levels of the brain chemical serotonin, which can also encourage feelings of hunger. So the cocktail of stress hormones plays with the delicate sensors in the reward centres of the brain, making unhealthy foods seem more rewarding and compellingly tasty.

Stress triggers a number of physiological mechanisms to give us the best chance of staying alive – these include increased heart rate to pump blood around the body, glucose flooding the bloodstream to give us energy, and pupil dilation to fine-tune vision so we can spot further danger. This made perfect sense to our hunter-gatherer ancestors because such physiological power-ups were vital if we were going to fight or flee a life-threatening predatory beast.

Today, this stress response can be helpful if it gets us out of the way of a swerving car, for instance, but it is not healthy long-term. When the stress response is switched on, other important functions are switched off, such as those involved with the immune system and effective digestion.

After a stressful outburst our bodies are very good at returning to a resting state thanks to the parasympathetic nervous system, which works as a relaxing counter to the stress-triggered sympathetic nervous system. This is known as a state of 'rest and digest' as the autonomic nervous system kick-starts any abandoned functions again.

But if we find ourselves in a constant state of stress (which is very common in today's world), your poor body doesn't get a break. Stress hormones like adrenaline and cortisol might be fantastic for short-term survival, but long term they can make weight loss tricky. One reason is the fact that our stress response floods the blood with glucose (emergency 'fight or flight' fuel). When we don't fight or flee, insulin is pumped out to move this extra glucose out of the blood and into fat cells. Stress triggers the laying down of fat.

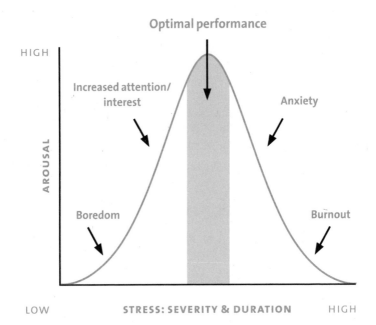

It also makes us chose unhealthy foods. Scans show that stress activates certain areas of the brain at the cost of the areas involved in executive function and cognitive reasoning, processes that are fundamental to decision making.[34][35] Researchers have found when people are in a highly stressful situation, they make less rational and practical decisions,[36] particularly in emotionally laden contexts.[37] On average, we make 221 food decisions each day, most of them completely outside our conscious awareness.[38] With this many food choices to make each day, and busy, sometimes stressful lives, stress will certainly be guiding some of the decisions about what and how much we eat.

You could be bored

Stress isn't always bad. We need it to get us motivated and out of bed in the morning and without that kind of stimulation, boredom can set in – and being bored can lead to grazing and weight gain.[39]

Just like Goldilocks and her bowls of porridge, too little or too much arousal from stress is not ideal (see graph opposite). Under-arousal can be caused by habituation which happens when the environmental stimuli around us are unchanging and unchallenging. Without enough stimulation or minds can wander and become preoccupied with thoughts of food and eating. However, too much pressure and stress (bearing in mind we all differ in our tolerance for demands) can result in feelings of anxiety that may lead us to turn to food as an escape or as a way of balancing stress hormones. The key is finding a balance between stimulation and feeling over-whelmed. If you've ever found yourself zombie-eating a pack of biscuits while finishing a tedious report, you're not the only one.

The Shrinktastic Twist

You may be surprised to see how many of the factors in this chapter apply to you. It is quite remarkable how our body and brain learn to cope with the pressures of modern life, and the extent to which adaptations like these conspire to make dieting and weight loss so supremely difficult.

Whether you could relate to one, a few, or to all of the possible factors we have outlined, these, in combination, help form the foundations of the way you behave when it comes to food and eating – very often without you even realising. They also form a constituent part of what makes up your Shrinkology type. You'll find personalised solutions to these problems, specific to the way they affect you and hold you back from your weight loss goals in Part Three.

Chapter 2
The Power of 'Big Food'

We live in a world where it is desirable to be slim, yet we are surrounded by food and bombarded by clever food marketing. It is hardly surprising that so many of us develop a difficult relationship with food that makes dieting seem impossible.

Not only are our bodies subconsciously conspiring against us to make weight gain seemingly inevitable, but the food industry, and the sometimes insidious power of social media, is adding immeasurably to the pressure many of us feel to eat unhealthily, in too-large quantities, and too often.

According to US biochemist, Dr Stephan Guyenet, under most conditions, your brain's energy-balance system should be highly effective, balancing your food consumption against your activity levels to ensure you stay at a healthy weight. When it is working best, this should be achieving 99.5 per cent accuracy in matching calories in vs calories out, thereby keeping you at a steady healthy weight.

But the brain's function is strongly challenged by the constant pressures on our natural reward system. For our ancestors, killing a large animal or finding a nest full of honey was a rare and wonderful event, so it made sense to overeat at those moments and store as many calories as possible for the lean times that might come later.[40]

Now, however, there's a veritable nest of honey on every street corner and a large animal already cut up and prepared in your fridge and freezer. This excessive availability triggers an 'evolutionary mismatch'. With easy access and delicious food readily available, overeating is inevitable and difficult to counter.

Food shops are open through the night and apps can deliver takeaways to your door at the touch of a button. This is not how we evolved to thrive. Dr Guyenet says that this means the slow, rational decision-making part of our brain can become kicked into touch by the fast, intuitive non-conscious part that is more likely to grab food without really thinking. This process is what so often undermines our good intentions, and ensures, he says, that we now typically eat around 200 calories per day more than we did in 1975.

There are plenty of studies to back up this theory. Some show that mice allowed to eat whenever they like (day and night) gain more weight than those eating during an eight-hour window, even when both are fed the same high-fat diet.[41] Epidemiologists at Cambridge University tracked more than 5,000 workers, looking at their consumption of and exposure to takeaway food. They found that greater access to takeaway food was linked with higher odds of obesity, with those most exposed to takeaway food outlets nearly twice as likely to be obese.[42]

If you've ever popped into a supermarket for milk and emerged with a bag of goodies you hadn't intended to buy, or found yourself somehow holding a chocolate bar as you queue to pay for fuel at the filling station (though you went in with no intention to do so), agreed to a sack of popcorn with your cinema tickets or tucked into a packet of crisps with your glass of wine, you'll know you've been 'had' by marketing. You have fallen into the food companies' clever trap: paying to buy food items that you don't really want or need. It's money in the bank for them and unnecessary calories for you.

The food industry spends millions of pounds in food development, packaging and marketing to find new and better ways to persuade you to eat more than you want or need. What chance has even the strongest willpower got against this multi-million pound marketing muscle?

In the last decade, an increasing number of scientists have attempted to stand up to the big food companies, calling on them to take some responsibility for a contributing role in fuelling the worldwide obesity epidemic. Many are likening the seriousness of the situation to that faced by the tobacco industry. The health hazards of smoking were known in the mid-1950s, yet tobacco companies continued to aggressively market cigarettes using sporting figures and ads portraying doctors, dentists and scientists in their attempt to give an air of implied healthiness. First, they issued an ad (in 1954) to counter reports that smoking cigarettes could cause lung cancer and had other dangerous health effects. But they started to add filter tips to remove some of the tar and nicotine, and 'safer' brands were introduced. By 2004, sales of 'light' cigarettes had overtaken conventional cigarette sales.

Sound familiar? The food industry is as determined (if not more so) to beat the nay-sayers and get straight to your purse. In 1990, Coca-Cola allegedly set a sales goal much larger than merely beating the rival brands – a senior executive revealed it strove to outsell every other thing people drank, including milk and water. Its goals have since publicly changed, to a more outwardly healthy focus on providing consumers with more low- or no-calorie products – but still products from which they can profit.[43]

Light cigarettes, diet drinks … can you see the trend?

Like the tobacco companies before them, the food industry has a dedicated, financially and politically powerful strategy to deflect the responsibility and blame for the obesity epidemic on to the individual. It's not *their* fault you are struggling with your weight – we are all clearly eating too much and exercising too little, they say. And, as a show of good faith, many have been developing and marketing 'healthy' diet foods and sponsoring big sporting events (see below) to inspire us all to be more active.

Yale University Professor of Psychology and Public Health, Kelly Brownell, is one of many who believe the processed-food industry should be seen as a public health menace. She has said 'As a culture, we've become upset by the tobacco companies advertising to children, but we sit idly by while the food companies do the very same thing. And we could make a claim that the toll taken on the public health by a poor diet rivals that taken by tobacco.'

In 2012, lawyers in the US filed cases against food industry giants for misleading consumers with confusingly labelled products and ingredients. The response by 'big food' to growing criticism has been to argue that they are merely doing what the consumer wants. It is certainly true that they are not *forcing* you to buy doughnuts or burgers or pizza any more than tobacco companies would *force* you to smoke. But commerce is a dog-eat-dog world – if one big food producer holds back on chocolate chip cookies, stuffed crust pizzas or whipped cream lattes, a competitor will certainly step in to steal the market share.

There is an obvious clash between public health advocates and a powerful food lobby that will go to any length to protect their only interest: profit. The food industry is largely self-regulated, and, as public health expert Simon Capewell (Professor of Public Health and Policy at the University of Liverpool) said in 2012, allowing the food industry to self-regulate was 'like putting Dracula in charge of the blood bank'. That's how McDonald's and Coca-Cola ended up advocating the role of exercise in tackling obesity whilst using the Olympic Games, the most effective marketing platform in the world, to promote their brands.

Clever marketers know very well that we eat for many reasons as well as hunger. The first page of any food marketing manual will probably point out that food choice is influenced by a myriad of different factors such as concerns about health ('this looks healthy'), mood ('this might cheer me up'), pure convenience ('it's quick and transportable'), sensory appeal (crunch, melt in the mouth, sweet, salt, etc.), natural content ('ah! Organic! It must be good'), price ('such good value!'), weight control ('it's low-fat so it will help me lose weight'), familiarity ('this is a brand I can trust'), and some-times ethical concern.[44]

We might not be able to avoid the power of 'big food', but we can adopt a Shrinkology mindset and empower ourselves by under-standing a little bit about how we are being manipulated by very clever people expert in ways to bamboozle a healthy eating mindset and instigate mindless grazing.

Why does junk food taste so good?

Not content with just marketing food to make it irresistible, over recent decades big food companies have also become wonderfully adept at making food addictive (or at least highly compelling), convenient and inexpensive (which means profitable).

The grandmaster of taste manipulation in recent years has been a man called Howard Moskowitz, a US experimental psychologist whose first job straight out of college in the 1970s was working on a mission for the US Army to persuade soldiers to eat more rations in the field. The Army was concerned that soldiers found their meals so boring they'd throw them away half eaten and not consume the calories they needed.

Moskowitz very cleverly identified the concept of 'sensory-specific satiety' which explains how adding big, distinct flavours doesn't tempt us to eat more, but can have the opposite effect, over-whelming the brain and actually depressing your desire to have more. They key, he found, was to create foods with the perfect balance of flavour combinations to 'trick' the soldiers' brains and ensure they continued to eat whether they were hungry or not.

It's a theory which might have been revelatory for the US Army, and ultimately beneficial for hard-working soldiers, and today, sensory-specific satiety remains a guiding principle for the processed-food industry – but it's not so good for us.

Food scientists since have found that manipulating flavour and texture like this can create 'hyperpalatability'. Processed foods are often engineered to have complex flavour combinations that create an almost never-ending satiety loop. Many packaged goods are dosed with immense amounts of refined sweeteners and salt, which, when eaten regularly, dull your taste buds, meaning you require ever-increasing levels of flavour to achieve the same taste satisfaction.

The biggest food and drink hits of all time – be they Coca-Cola or Doritos – owe their success to complex formulas that pique the taste buds enough to be alluring without having a distinct, over-riding single flavour that tells the brain to stop eating. The most difficult foods to resist are those with complex flavours (sweet and salty like salted caramel) because the brain takes longer to register 'taste satiety' over multiple tastes.

In fact, Howard Moskowitz coined the term 'Bliss Point' to define the perfect balance of salt/sweet/fat which has been found to 'opti-mise palatability' and create the greatest amount of 'crave'. He described it as 'that sensory profile where you like the food the most'. Studies show that sugar, fat and salt act synergistically together, giving a stronger sense of reward than alone. Think crisps, and salted caramel. That's obvious. But it also explains why sugar is now added routinely to processed savoury foods (ketchup, soups, pizzas, ready meals, sauces) to engineer a more potent bliss point.

NOT JUST HUMANS

This isn't just theoretical: studies show the best way to fatten a rat is to feed it human food – it will ignore all satiety signals and just keep eating. That's why the Shrinkology Solution advocates the eating of real, not processed food. Give your brain the best chance to make satiety decisions for itself.

Snacking is a relatively recent concept and one that has been created and fuelled by profit-driven food companies for profit. Right up until the 1970s, your standard snack was a piece of fruit, or possibly a biscuit, and the chocolate bar Milky Way was advertised as something 'you can eat between meals without ruining your appetite'. This is a gentle marketing approach that now looks rather quaint.

Today, marketing reports indicate that snacking is the biggest food growth area, with 94 per cent of us snacking once a day and one in four 'super-snackers' snacking four or more times a day.

Every new processed snack food is devised by food scientists to be a bite-sized delight which hits that super-profitable bliss point. It's a hugely lucrative business which has spawned the invention of cereal bars, energy balls, Pop-Tarts, Lunchables, Pringles, pizza chips, Fruit Winders …

It is marketing genius, and it is one big reason why so many of us are struggling to control our weight. If we snacked only occasionally, and in small amounts, this would not present the enormous problem that it does. But because so much money and effort have been invested over decades in engineering and then relentlessly selling these products, the effects are seemingly impossible to unwind.

In most cases, meals are just meals at their most basic level, but snacks have been very cleverly designed and packaged to help *define* their purchaser. Yes, you might buy a certain brand of bread or breakfast cereal because it fits your values (healthy/indulgent/ostentatious) but that has limited public display appeal. Most of the consumption will be behind closed doors. But snacks are carried and displayed, eaten or drunk in public. To many, they are all part of an image that must be nurtured and upheld. Your snack of choice will be carefully selected to reflect and endorse a certain style or personality.

The snacking marketing culture *feeds* the distorted behaviour that leads to disordered eating. Marketing literature helpfully points out that snacking 'occasions' can be early morning, mid-morning, lunch, mid-afternoon, evening, late at night. Nourishment is only one defined snacking 'need' – the true concern is profit dressed up by the food industry as 'satisfaction of craving', relaxation and reward. How much more profitable it is to create a snack that not only satisfies a craving, but also creates a craving at the same time – thereby doubling your purchasing potential?

The Shrinkology solution is simple. Don't snack. Stop buying snacks. Eat meals instead, and if you get caught out hungry, just wait a little. You can do this.

Why is chocolate so delicious?

Chocolate is food design genius and perfect for overriding hunger signals. The sugar and fat combination closely mimics that of breast milk (so drawing us to memories of comfort we will have long forgotten) and it has a 33.8 degrees Celsius melting point, which is just slightly cooler than body temperature (37 degrees Celsius) meaning it feels cold on the tongue, then slowly melts . . . Studies show that letting chocolate dissolve slowly in your mouth can produce as big an increase in brain activity and heart rate as a passionate kiss.

The several hundred different plant chemicals in cocoa also combine to create the taste sensation, but that's not all. Researchers at the Neurosciences Institute in San Diego, California, say chocolate contains a feel-good chemical called anandamide which is found naturally in the brain, and is similar to a substance found in marijuana. Normally anandamide is broken down quite quickly after it is produced, but the San Diego chemists think the anandamide in chocolate makes the natural anandamide in our brain persist for longer – in other words, it gives us a longer-lasting 'chocolate high'.[45] The impact of all this really *is* more intense if you are a chocoholic. In 2007 Oxford University psychologists compared brain scans of people eating chocolate and found self-confessed chocoholics had increased action in parts of the brain that tend to be involved in addictive behaviour – they found looking at pictures of chocolate triggered the same impact as eating it.[46]

The good news for chocoholics is you should get the same chemical 'kick' from really dark chocolate as white, and that bitter confection has much less sugar and fewer calories, with a really intensive propensity for your chocolate high. You might need to wean yourself down slowly by gradually increasing cocoa solid percentages as your taste buds become accustomed to less sugar and fat, but it means you can still enjoy chocolate without guilt or self-recrimination.

Beware the Diet Industry

You'd think the very lucrative diet industry would have our best interests at heart, wouldn't you? Surely diet drinks help you slim, meal replacements offer wholesome calorie-counted options to real food, and 'low-fat' or 'no-added-sugar' options are much healthier than their full-fat and sugar-enhanced predecessors? Sadly not. If diet foods worked, diet food companies would rapidly go out of business.

We have to be realistic about the commercial realities here. The diet industry is a multi-million pound, highly profitable business and its long-term success depends upon you losing *just* enough weight to continue, but not so much that you don't keep coming back for more. Its profitability depends on our human failings and successfully exploiting them.

The big drinks companies are wealthy enough to pump millions into sponsorship deals and advertising campaigns, so you'd think they'd be able to support research to back up a belief that diet drinks aid weight loss? Sadly, no such evidence exists. Some scientists increasingly believe that many artificial sweeteners might provide you with a 'zero calorie' product, but they confuse the delicate balance of chemicals in the body and the brain, which could lead you to eat *more* not less.

All too often a 'low-fat' or 'reduced-fat' food will be pumped with extra sugar, sweeteners and clever chemical compounds to compensate for the taste and 'mouth feel' that fat normally provides. Far from being healthier or better for you, these foods are just chemically altered in such a way to make you keep on buying them in the hope that they'll help you lose weight.

This is true at the other end of the scale, too: highly processed foods are often packed with cheap ingredients, regardless of how they're marketed. Often, processing food means removing fibre, such as in white bread, rice and pasta. This increases that food's calorie density and makes that food so much easier to overeat. Though highly tempting, and sometimes delicious, processed foods, whether high-fat and high-sugar 'treat' foods (doughnuts, crisps, cakes and biscuits) or low fat and low-sugar 'diet' foods interfere with some of the ways our natural energy-balance system senses that we've had enough. Studies show we tend to eat more when a food is called 'healthy'– not just more of the 'healthy' food, but more food generally, without feeling guilty.[47] It seems the 'healthy' food casts a healthy glow over all our eating behaviours, negating any extra calories in our mind.[48] [49]

In fact, even merely thinking about picking a healthier option without actually consuming it can be enough to somehow trick you into thinking you're being healthy, which can make you feel hungrier and entice you to choose the most indulgent food available.[50] [51]

Shrewd labelling is all part of the food marketing subterfuge. A box of cereal might cleverly avoid a 'red light' for sugar content by stating per-portion amounts for the tiny bowlful you'd give a child. You could be tucking into a moderately sized adult portion without realising you are busting healthy limits.

Food companies are obliged to state the ingredients in order of weight, so to maintain a 'healthy' status, they'll cleverly sub-divide sugar into different types (honey, maple syrup, dextrose, cane sugar, corn syrup, fructose ...), each of which can be listed separately and in smaller quantities, which allows them to be lined up at the back of the queue, but they are all still sugar!

In your quest to become truly Shrinktastic, you're going to have to learn to apply a delicious dollop of healthy cynicism to processed foods – no matter what 'low-fat, low-sugar' claims are being made on the label – and start to embrace real food, rather than diet food.

Could social media be affecting your weight?

We are constantly bombarded by 'ideal' images in newspapers, magazines, on TV and especially online. Logically we know many of these images are teased and stretched, doctored and Photoshopped. Public image is all about lighting, angles and selection. But our subconscious mind remains gullible, and it can be a struggle not to compare those images to what we see in the mirror every day and end up feeling dissatisfied.

So many girls grow up into women who can't shake off the ideal image of 'thin as beautiful'. It's clearly not healthy. Psychologists know that internalising a thin ideal leads to us becoming unhappy with ourselves and this can in turn generate unhelpful views towards food and eating, in particular dieting. For decades, news-papers and magazines were blamed for publishing pictures of rake-thin models perpetuating an impossibly skinny ideal. But you can multiply that exposure exponentially if you're a keen social media addict, spending hours each day flicking through perfection on your phone.

You might think you're just being nosy and voyeuristic as you scroll through the Kardashian Insta feed, or rush to catch up with Victoria Beckham, but this constant stream of unattainable (and very often airbrushed) beauty is definitely not good for your mental health. Social media makes it so hard to be happy with your body and your weight, and so hard to achieve a happy, healthy weight.

There's also the culture of Photoshopped perfection that massively amplifies body dissatisfaction[52] feeding the diet business. 'Clean eating' bloggers rarely mention weight loss, but their ethos can sometimes hide a desire for thinness and sculpted, self-conscious beauty, all to be achieved seemingly without effort. But this aspirational slenderness is hard to achieve and not really very different from the rejected old-fashioned diets of restriction.

It's not only women who feel and bend to this pressure. Men are also influenced by advertising[53] – if they weren't then there wouldn't be such astronomical budgets for ad slots in sporting events. However, for men, thinness is combined with muscle definition to create that difficult-to-achieve, six-pack ideal. Researchers at Harvard Medical School have identified a condition called 'muscle belittlement' whereby men think they're less muscular than they really are. This distorted belief is thought to lie behind unhealthy eating patterns, use of performance-enhancing substances (muscle-building supplements and even steroids), low self-esteem and, in extreme cases, depression.[54]

Today, social media invades almost every aspect of our lives. It's no longer a young person's pastime – Instagram, Twitter, Facebook and Pinterest are compelling and compulsive essential accessories to almost every career and hobby. Yes, social media can bring joy and friendship. But it can also be very destructive and frighteningly addictive. Studies now show that the more time you spend sharing, liking, tweeting and hash-tagging, the greater your risk of unhappiness is likely to be.[55]

Too much exposure to social media, whether its old-fashioned celebrities or the new breed of foodie influencer, can distract from the real reasons to eat and what to eat. You might think you're in complete control, but the association between the beautiful, seemingly happy and perfect individuals on social media platforms with the food they are presenting can be utterly compelling. It can lead us to believe that if only we cooked and ate exactly what these Insta-celebs do, we too could be happy and life would be a breeze. Social media food fads, which make food a fashion item, create yet another pressure on us. This elevates food way beyond its original status as a source of sustenance, and creates desire wrapped up in an ever-changing fashion buzz we struggle to keep up with. This can leave us feeling like we're never quite good enough, and this can lead to body dissatisfaction. In some cases body dysmorphia can result, if someone becomes so obsessive about areas of their body that they spend an inordinate amount of time worrying about perceived imperfections that no one else can even see.

That sense of competition with others to get the most friends, followers or likes, coupled with the temptation to derive self-worth from how many comments and shares your posts receive, could be breeding a dependence on external sources of validation that leaves us feeling bad about ourselves when no one acknowledges a post they were hoping to get a huge response from. Social media can be isolating and, ironically, can make you feel disconnected and alone. These feelings can often result in social anxiety. Stress increases cortisol levels, which we know can be fattening for some people.

BE SHRINKTASTIC ABOUT SOCIAL MEDIA

One important tenet of the Shrinkology Solution is to throw a lasso around your social media use and ask yourself whether everything on your social media feed is truly helpful. Be realistic, be Shrinktastic, work out ways to trim some of the fat and instead refresh your feed with inspirational and healthy sources which motivate you to exercise and offer deliciously healthy recipe ideas instead. Find and follow the sort of influencers more likely to make you feel strong and empowered, and choose to surround yourself with positive healthy eating messages for the times when you are checking your phone.

At the end of the day, there's a lot to be said for taking regular social media breaks – you could even switch off completely for a while. Check out the social media controlling/corralling tips designed to really hit the button for each Shrinkology type.

Ultimately, constantly comparing ourselves to airbrushed images leads to body dissatisfaction, which in turn is linked to overeating and/or cycles of eating and dieting.

And it isn't just about people. Glossy pictures of appetising food or cooking have long been used by the advertising industry to tempt us to eat more, and such is the social media seduction that 'food porn' now even has its own searchable hashtag. If you choose to fill your social media feed with these delicious images, you might notice a change in your waistline.

Regularly viewing mouthwatering food photos on social media may trigger feelings of hunger and encourage overindulgence.

Studies show that looking at pictures of food is enough to raise a person's levels of ghrelin, a hormone involved in the stimulation of hunger, as the tasty image sends a rush of blood to the part of the brain responsible for taste, encouraging you to eat, even when you're not hungry. Researchers call this 'visual hunger'[56] and it applies to cookery shows and flicking through recipe books.[57] It certainly helps explain why it's so hard to watch *Bake Off* without reaching for a biscuit or a slice of cake.

The Shrinktastic Twist

Food science, advertising and marketing have become a highly specialised force which very cleverly tempts us to buy and consume food we might not really want or need. We'd be mad to underestimate its power. This effect is magnified by the inexorable rise of social media. Together, these additional pressures subtly persuade us that what we eat and our body shape and size define us. Understanding these forces is the next step in your Shrinkology awareness journey.

Once you are fully aware of these influences on your eating behaviour, you'll be in the best place to start making profound, lasting shifts in your life that can free you from the shackles of body dissatisfaction and perpetual yo-yo dieting.

Chapter 3
You Can Change your Behaviour, Long Term

It is clear that numerous outside forces conspire to influence your eating behaviour, and everyone responds differently.

But the really important message is that your individual dietary peccadilloes – whether you can't walk past a burger bar without popping in, whether one biscuit means you'll eat the whole packet, whether you struggle to function without four diet colas a day or you secretly swig double cream from the fridge – are just the surface manifestation of these influences. They are the symptom rather than the root cause of your dissatisfaction with your weight. As any gardener knows, chopping off the visible surface weeds will not stop them growing back. Random attempts at dieting don't work: you need to tackle the roots. That's where Shrinkology comes in.

The key to the Shrinkology Solution is believing that you have the power to change your life. It is so very easy to fall into an easy pattern of acceptance and convince yourself that your fate and your weight are out of your control or merely down to chance or a genetic or circumstantial lottery. But numerous studies have shown that anyone and everyone can acquire the necessary self-belief to make lasting positive changes – you just have to start with bite-sized, achievable mini goals.

The big stumbling block when you hitch yourself to a seemingly insurmountable global health aim like 'I must be fitter/slimmer/ healthier' is that although there are plenty of diet and exercise plans, until now there's been no proper mental roadmap to help you navigate your way through the complex emotional and behavioural patterns that govern the way you live your life. Shrinkology is your key to creating a truly personalised and effective plan. This book is your satnav on the journey to a long-term healthy weight without constant ineffectual dieting. Not everyone who has a genetic predisposition to weight gain was rewarded with food as a child, and not everyone who finds themselves struggling through an impossibly stressful life finds maintaining an optimal weight difficult, demonstrating that *all* of these factors can be overcome – yes, *all*, even including inheriting a 'fat gene'! In the face of all the formidable and persuasive pressures to consume energy-dense foods that we outlined earlier, resilience is absolutely key. And the good news? Resilience really can be nurtured and grown from within. The first step is understanding that unwelcome weight gain is probably *not your fault*, and *you do have the power* to change it.

Resilience is not about effortlessly bouncing back from adversity, but rather making best use of a set of new tools to evolve and adjust, and create a truly personalised approach to managing some of the most challenging aspects of your life. This, your Shrinkology toolkit, is key to effortless weight maintenance and, once established, it will stay with you long into the future even if the going gets tougher than it is right now.

You CAN rewire your brain

Scientists used to think that the brain was hard-wired at key developmental phases throughout your life – for instance when we first establish our caregiver attachment (see page 27). During this period the environment was thought to have a strong influence, which is why early life experiences are seen to be particularly important to us. But now we know that this isn't so simple – new networks can be built in our brains, allowing for further learning and habit changing, something called 'brain plasticity', or neuroplasticity. This means that even associations you might have learned many years ago, and which might have doggedly persisted through to adulthood, can be updated at any time.

It's similar to organising a software update for your computer. By trying new things, you can strengthen the connections between neurons and make new connections but also allow old, now unwanted associations to die off. You may have known every country's capital when you were at school and needed this knowledge for your geography exam, but after 30 years of *not* thinking about these facts, can you still remember them all? Likely a few, but it will be hard work – the neural connections have loosened over time, and the same can happen with eating habits.

This is incredibly important to realise because even after reading Chapter 1 you might worry that you could be stuck, or trapped, in the status quo (such as eating what your parents ate and the foods you liked as a child). You really don't have to be. But any new association requires considerable repetition (it takes time to learn something new) and changing, altering or improving pathways and associations will take repetition and practice.

It might seem hard to train yourself to eat at a slower pace, not in front of the TV and not with a glass of wine in hand, but by acting out these new eating behaviours over and over again, you can strengthen the new neural networks. In each of the type chapters, you'll find a wonderful assortment of expert mind hacks to help. Think of these as new skills to try, cherry pick and customise so they work perfectly for you. When it comes to the brain, practice really does make perfect.

The hacks will not only help you to alter your relationship with food and eating, but they will help in numerous other areas of life.

Studies repeatedly show these hacks work, and they are key to putting you fundamentally in control of your thought patterns and emotions to ensure you are less vulnerable to everyday stresses – in fact they could give you a whole new perspective on life.

And it isn't just about your brain. We now know that even if someone has a particular gene – say the fat gene – the volume dial on this gene and the extent to which it affects you, and the way you live your life, can be turned down or ramped up. You might still have that gene buried away deep inside your DNA, but the way your cells read the DNA sequence really can be altered by your behaviour. This means that having the fat gene isn't a *fait accompli* at all, as so much of what we do on a daily basis can influence this gene expression. So the food we eat, the sorts of exercise we do (or if we do none at all), whether we get enough good-quality sleep, and the speed at which we age, are all factors which play into influencing how your genes 'express' themselves.[58]

Although it's hard to change long-established eating patterns, particularly if they have served you well for many years, it *is* possible. Many vegetarians and vegans still crave meat and dairy products but can successfully eat in line with their strongly held beliefs. We can all alter our eating preferences at will when it is demanded (a family meal, dinner with the boss) and so, when it suits us, we can all override cravings. We just need to change when we decide to do so.

You CAN beat cravings

Sometimes when the thought of chocolate pops into your mind, or you pick up a chilled glass of wine and just can't stop believing it would taste so much better if matched with the satisfying crunch of a salty crisp, it can feel as if cravings are overwhelming. They can certainly be all-consuming!

But from a psychological perspective, cravings are short – they rarely last more than three minutes and just knowing this and, crucially, believing it, can help you feel more in control and help you overcome them. Distracting your attention away from a craving for a short time really can help it pass. In Part Three you'll find clever cravings-busting tips individually targeted for your Shrinkology type.

Whatever your type, you can boost your cravings-busting effectiveness with a few strategic moves to protect and preserve your willpower throughout the day. Just as any muscle in your body might start to get tired at the end of a long day, so your willpower is vulnerable to fatigue.[59] If you know you have to face a full-on, stress-packed day that will deplete your willpower reserves (you'll use up some willpower trying not to tell your boss what you really think, a little more trying to be polite to an incredibly rude co-worker, more still fighting the urge to lay your head on the table after lunch for a quick snooze ...) don't make this a fasting day of hardcore food restriction. Self-control requires a certain amount of calorific energy and if your petrol tank is running low you will find it harder to say 'no thanks' to the dessert menu.[60] The fast-depleting willpower pot also means if you're facing a tricky challenge, aim to do it in the morning rather than late at night when your willpower has packed up for the evening and left you at the mercy of your conscience.

You CAN take control of your thoughts

Our thoughts have a big influence on our behaviour – this is why psychological therapies such as cognitive behaviour therapy (CBT; see page 172) have been so successfully used to help people cope with chronic pain, social anxiety and insomnia. So even if in your darkest moments you wonder whether you'd be more successful, popular or content if you were happier with your weight, you do face a choice – you can choose to completely reject the prevailing notion that weight and worth are invariably tied together.

The first and significant step is learning to accept that there are tremendous forces trying to make us feel bad about the way we look in order to sell us not only diet products but perfume, fashion, skin-care and many other big ticket items that we don't particularly need.

You can choose instead to focus on how you *feel*. It is within your power. For sure, feeling strong, energetic, calm, grounded and engaged with others is a healthier focus than driving yourself crazy over whether the numbers on your bathroom scales are going up or down.

You need to know and to believe that the dieting industry has been created not only to meet a need, but also, conveniently, to generate a need. By perpetuating the stereotype that thinness equals happiness rather than celebrating the wide range of different body shapes and sizes, this hugely lucrative industry can keep churning out profits.

Learning to cultivate a degree of self-acceptance is the best way to allow you to let go of perfectionist and unrealistic views of the physical body. Just think of how much time and headspace you'd have if you weren't thinking about food and dieting for such a large part of every day. Self-acceptance is the key to a long-term, healthy body and you'll find type-specific hacks and exercises to try in Part Three.

You CAN live in the here and now

If we let ourselves mull over the past or allow a constant negative chatter about the future to run through our minds we are not living properly or effectively in the present. Not only does this fill your headspace with an unnecessary amount of negativity but it stops you being able to fully enjoy what you've already got. Learning how to bring your focus back to the 'here and now' can have a myriad of health benefits, over and above weight loss. Shrinkology will show you how.

You CAN take the red pill

In the film *The Matrix*, the central character Neo (played by Keanu Reeves) is offered the choice of taking a blue pill or a red pill. He is told the blue pill will keep him in blissful ignorance in a dream world that is safe, comfortable and familiar but also secretly a form of enslavement. The red pill, on the other hand, will wake him up from this dream and dump him into a much harsher and more dangerous reality. It might be tough, but in red pill land, Neo has the potential to influence his own destiny.

The blue pill represents security in what you already know, even if it's untrue, whereas the red pill represents the reality achieved through knowledge and the surety that with that knowledge comes freedom.

You are going to be in your body for the rest of your life – being happy about your body and your weight is very much part of the long game. Although dieting can be effective,[61] your success – or not – will depend on your perception of where you've been, where you're at and where you're going.

Most restrictive diets offer little more than a short-term, sticking plaster fix. If you want to put an end to the relentless and tedious round of yo-yo dieting, you need to stop taking that particular blue pill. *The Shrinkology Solution* is your red pill. Thankfully it is not harsh, dangerous or tough, but it does require a fresh new approach and a commitment to making long-term changes to your diet and your attitudes towards food that you can stick with for the rest of your life.

Part Two
Become Your Own Shrinkologist

In this section, we bring together key principles of psychology to outline the importance of creating your own food and mood diary (chapter 4). This will help you pinpoint your individual emotional and behavioural characteristics around food. You can then feed these findings into the Shrinkology Quiz (chapter 5) to discover your dominant Shrinkology Type. Before you turn to Part Three and start building your personalised Shrinkology Solution, it's time to embrace a few Shrinkology Fundamentals (chapter 6) which will form the strong foundations for a new, long-lasting, healthy relationship with food.

Chapter 4
Shrinkology Diagnostics

Taking a Shrinkology approach to sustained and steady long-term weight maintenance is all about understanding your own personal triggers, weaknesses and influences when it comes to food, drilling down and coming up with your own Shrinkology diagnosis.

The first step in the Shrinkology process is make a commitment to change. Numerous studies have shown that making a firm commitment to change can really boost your mood and provide the catalyst you need to make changes stick.[62]

Once you have committed to change, the next step is creating your own personalised food/mood diary. This is a really powerful diagnostic tool. It is the next important step in personalising your Shrinkology Solution and the best possible way to help you better understand your eating triggers and behavioural patterns when it comes to food, and what's more, it will help you to diagnose your type as accurately as possible.

Done properly, a food/mood diary will really open your eyes to every aspect of your relationship with food and how this impacts on the way you eat. It is the best possible way to uncover emotional eating patterns and identify triggers that might prompt overeating.

HOW TO INTENSIFY YOUR COMMITMENT:

- Tell others about your planned health changes. Not only will the support of close friends and family help you to keep on track, you may well inspire them to make positive changes too.
- Write down reminders of your commitment to change. Stick them on the fridge, on the home page of your mobile phone or computer, so you will look at them every day. Simple visual prompts can be powerful aids to maintaining a health change.
- Celebrate every small success either with non-food treats, by sharing your success with others or by noting each accomplishment in a journal.

TACKLE ANY BUTS:

If there are any 'buts' lurking, tackle them now by thinking up strong counter arguments of your own:
- But I'm not sure if I will be 'me' if I change my eating patterns;
- But I don't think my family will want to eat my new diet so it will be hard;
- But I can't afford to buy expensive healthy ingredients;
- But I don't have time to cook at home.

Before you start, make sure you have strong, clear answers for any buts, so you are prepared to fight them when they creep into your mind.

A food/mood diary works by making you fully aware of what, how much, and why you are eating. It's a great way to highlight not just the foods you might not usually notice yourself nibbling but specifically why you are eating them (and, if you're reading this book, there's every chance that for you, hunger isn't always a factor).

Studies show that when people complete any type of food diary or activity journal, they're very often shocked to see the reality of their eating behaviours. Because, as we have seen, eating is only partially about hunger, and very often our overt eating behaviour is simply the tip of the iceberg. Your diary is a powerful weight-loss and weight-maintenance tool. Studies show dieters who make a note of everything they eat and how much exercise they do can lose twice as much weight as those who don't.[63] [64] In fact, diet experts believe keeping a very careful food diary could help you lose three times as much weight as not keeping a diary at all.

Very often, the prospect of having to write 'four chips from partner's plate' or 'snatched handful of peanuts' is enough to stop you from mindlessly reaching out for unhealthy foods in the first place, and it's too easy to 'forget' about that nibbled biscuit, or underestimate the size of your bowl of cereal if you leave your diary entries until the end of each day.

Not only will this diary guide you and help you be conscientious, it will show up patterns (does a certain kind of breakfast leave you hungry mid-morning? Are your cravings worse at times high stress?), which will give you an insight into the helpful, healthy habits you can develop in Part Three.

Social gatherings can highjack all efforts at reasonable eating, so do jot this down in your diary too. Social triggers prove that the link between food and mood isn't just a negative one – feeling excited and celebratory can lead to mindless eating and drinking. Your diary might expose a string of unknown associations between particular friends or family members and eating behaviours e.g. you always have a bottle of wine when seeing a best mate. Some patterns might be life-affirming, but others could be unhelpful. You'll find lots of solutions in your Shrinkology type chapter.

The key is carrying your diary with you at all times and writing down absolutely *everything* that goes in your mouth the moment it happens – and your mood before and afterwards. Be absolutely honest with your entries. You're doing this for yourself – so *no cheating!* Even if you find yourself finishing off a whole packet of biscuits, jot this down in your diary. Make a note of the circumstances and your feelings too. Were you feeling hungry? Hormonal? Lonely? Bored? Stressed? Having these notes when you look back over your week can give you invaluable pointers about your emotional state, which will help you make the most of the tips to suit your Shrinkology type, and so effectively work to avoid these situations in the future.

For best results, keep your diary going every day, for at least one week (preferably more). It can be very tempting to relax at the weekends, but for many people weekends are the most important days to keep tabs on food intake, because a weekend represents 28.57% of your week and is when many people let their good intentions slip, meaning you can easily lose a third of your week's hard work.

TAKE IT ONLINE

Look out for the latest apps which might make logging your food and mood more immediat. A study found that participants who monitored their diet with either a smartphone app or memo feature missed fewer days of logging than people using paper and a pencil, possibly because apps are so easy to use.[65]

Check out RiseUp, FoodMood or Daylio.

Food diary

From the minute you wake up in the morning until you switch
off the light at night, track the following:

- what you eat or drink; and precisely how much you eat or drink
- what time you eat
- how much water are you drinking?
- how many portions of vegetables have you eaten? And how
  much fruit?
- how hungry were you before and after eating it – did you let
  yourself get too hungry before eating? Did you stop eating
  when you felt satisfied and no longer hungry, or full?
- when and how dramatic were any episodes of hunger or
  cravings, on a scale of 1 to 10?
- any food-related emotions/thoughts

Hunger scale

To help you get in tune with your body, rate your level
of hunger before and after each meal:

10 starving (weak, dizzy)
9 ravenous (irritable, low energy)
8 very hungry (stomach rumbling, preoccupied with food)
7 slightly hungry (thinking about food)
6 neutral
5 slightly full (pleasantly satisfied)
4 very full (uncomfortable)
3 stuffed (belt-loosening territory)
2 nauseous (painfully bloated and feeling sick)
1 medical attention (call a doctor!)

Make your diary work for you

At the end of the week sit down and review your food diary information. Ask yourself: what have you learned? Are there any clear patterns starting to form? You know by now there are many, many reasons *other* than hunger that drive us to eat. And your diary is a great way for you to start spotting patterns of eating behaviour.

On page 63, you'll find a handy tally table with the most common patterns of food behaviour. To use it, add a tick in your Shrinkology tally table each time you spot a behaviour in your diary which corresponds to a pattern in the table. Once you've completed the quiz, total the tallies on each column and find out which two behaviours have occurred most frequently. The letters in the columns respond to your Shrinkology type, so add these to the results of the quiz.

Don't worry if you have a scattering of ticks across the types. This is perfectly normal. But this information all feeds into a more finely tuned type diagnosis when you come to the quiz .

Patterns to look out for

Are you using foods to lift your mood?

Some foods really do have a direct impact on our mood by triggering the 'feel-good' neurotransmitters in our brain. We all vary in our sensitivity. Chocolate might trigger a noticeable boost in one person but not in another for whom the foil and paper wrapping signifies little more than a conveniently packaged source of energy.

When completing your food/mood diary it's important to note down not only how you feel *after* you eat or drink something, but *before* as well.

Researchers have found that in some people chocolate can act as an antidepressant,[66] for instance, and although supposedly 'healthy' drinks such as fruit smoothies might hike alertness (thanks to the fruit sugar they contain) they could leave you feeling jittery and

TIME	FOOD/DRINK	HUNGER LEVEL BEFORE & AFTER EATING (SEE GRID)	OTHER SYMPTOMS (e.g. STRESS, BOREDOM, CONCENTRATION DIFFICULTIES, ETC.)	FEELINGS/MOOD	WHAT WERE YOU DOING – WHERE, WITH WHOM?
06:34	Small glass of water	6/6	Tired, hard to get out of bed.	Dreading day, worried about work.	In bed, at home with partner.
07:11	Cup of tea, milk, 1 sugars/1 sweetener	8/8	Tummy rumbling, feel like can't do anything else now without food.	Stressed – mornings are always manic.	Getting kids up at home.
07:45	Cornflakes with semi-skimmed milk	10/5	Feeling sick and shaky.	Rather overwhelmed, feel like there's not enough time in the day.	Take kids to school, the in car to work at home, then out the door.
08:23	Milky coffee and pain au raisin	6/5		Feeling more relaxed now; 'me time' in car.	Stopped for petrol on way to work at car, alone.
10:05	Tea with milk (1 sugar/ 1 sweetener), 3 custard creams	5/5		Not feeling, focusing on meeting.	Working through weekly reports in board room with colleagues.

DAY	I USE FOODS TO LIFT MOOD C	I EAT TO ESCAPE C	I EAT TO DESTRESS F	I WORRY ABOUT WHAT I EAT B	I ALWAYS FINISH A PLATE OF FOOD D	I GIVE INTO CRAVINGS E
1						
2						
3						
4						
5						
6						
7						

DAY	I AM ALWAYS HUNGRY/SCARED TO BE HUNGRY A	INFREQUENT EATING F	FOOD CHOICES CAUSE STRESS B	I OVER-INDULGE AFTER BOOZE E	I'M A SOCIAL EATER A	I'M A HABITUAL EATER D
1						
2						
3						
4						
5						
6						
7						

over-excitable. This is commonly followed by a mood crash as the body tries to restore a sense of balance. If you notice this pattern, perhaps your meals are not giving you the sustained energy you need to get through the day (see Chapter 6, and investigate the tips and tricks in your type chapter for type-specific non-food ways to boost mood).

Do you eat to escape?

Sometimes we eat to dampen feelings that we perhaps don't want to feel. Eating can directly consume your focus so you can pretend to consciously ignore or fail to acknowledge deeper feelings. Or, interestingly, if you eat 'bad' food and feel subsequently guilty, you could be unconsciously using this 'food guilt' to mask other negative thoughts and feelings.

Sometimes it's easier to blame our 'uncontrolled' or 'ill-disciplined' eating and our unhappiness with our weight for why we feel dissatisfied or unfulfilled, when the true root could be something completely unrelated (such as early childhood experiences or a sense of loss, a relationship break-up or losing a connection with a friend). You need to be honest with yourself here and dig deep when completing your diary and looking at it afterwards – do cravings occur when other feelings are bubbling up?

Do you eat to destress?

Food can provide a wonderful distraction in times of stress. This actually has an evolutionary function – seeking out high-sugar, high-fat food may be an unconscious attempt by the brain to rebalance the levels of stress hormones, which in turn will dampen the stress response and unpleasant feeling of anxiety.[67] Long-term stress increases our risk of a raft of health problems, so the urge to eat comforting food may be our body's way of trying to rebalance.

Keep an eye out for these signs that might that indicate your stress levels are creeping up high:

PALPITATIONS: take note if your heart seems to skip a beat as this is often part of the flight-fight-freeze response.

WANDERING MIND: stress can affect your attention and ability to concentrate.

FIDGETING: restlessness can reflect your body's urge to escape from a stressful situation.

LOW LIBIDO: this is a common consequence of a demanding lifestyle, which can lead to extra stress.

STOMACH TROUBLE: the brain and gut communicate constantly, so the gut can tell you more about how you are feeling.

SLEEP PROBLEMS: these are linked to long-term stress – you shouldn't be able sleep with a lion (real or imagined) in the room, so if you're stressed the body won't let you.

IRREGULAR BREATHING: this often results in loss of or shaky voice, a sign to watch out for.

IRRITABILITY: a shorter fuse than usual is a common symptom of chronic stress, and could explain why you find you're snapping at family or losing patience with colleagues.

FEELING OVERWHELMED: if you sometimes feel you are sinking under the weight of the world, it might just be stress.

FREQUENT COUGHS AND COLDS: stress impairs the immune system. If you seem to pick up one thing after another or simply can't shake off a bug, your stress may have reached unsustainable levels.

Keep a close eye out for these signs, and if you spot them, be sure to make a note in your diary.

Your food/mood diary will help highlight the possibility that stress could have been part of your life for so long that you've just become accustomed to it. But there are so many things you can do to make your stress levels more manageable for your type, which will be covered in Part Three.

Are you worrying about what you eat?

Before you eat, have you spent a great deal of time deciding what to have, then feel overwhelmed by the choice? If you've been on and off diets for years, food can become a source of tension and concern as you run through your memory banks each time you put something in your mouth, to try to remember whether it's 'allowed' or not. Finding yourself concerned about your food choices can lead to erratic hunger patterns.

Do you scrape your plate clean even when you aren't hungry?

When looking at your hunger pre- and post-meal, are you ever painfully full? Did you finish a meal out of politeness? Or habit?

Are you succumbing to cravings?

If the urge to give in to foods – especially those that reach the bliss point – is overpowering, take a look at what you were doing before the craving. Can you identify anything useful in the circumstances related to craving cave-in?

Do you always seem to be hungry?

You could be eating erratically, making poor food choices, or are you eating because you're frightened of being *really* hungry? ('I'd better have a full meal now, even though I'm not really hungry, because it's a long time until my next meal.') Sometimes it is the fear of hunger not physical hunger driving eating behaviour, which could be related to food restriction in the past.

Are you eating infrequently?

Are you allowing lots of long gaps between meals? Are you actually eating enough? Do you go for hours and hours without eating and then find yourself uncontrollably stuffing your face because you're so hungry?

Do you eat/drink more when entertaining?

Are you a 'social eater'? We innately want to fit in, so the influence of others, even implicit peer pressure, can affect food intake. Booze is a killer for executive functions such as willpower and decision making, so keep an eye on how alcohol relates to food intake.

Have you developed some strong habitual eating links?

For example, having biscuits with tea, muffins with latte, crisps with wine, peanuts with beer ... Do you feel it's simply 'wrong' not to engage in these patterns?

You can also use the food/mood diary and tally table after you've discovered your Shrinkology type and started to use your personalised mind hacks and diet tips. By doing this you can track progress and identify any areas that still need attention. Nothing is more motivating than seeing change happen!

Chapter 5
What's your Shrinkology Type?

The next key step in your quest to create a truly personalised Shrinkology solution is discovering which Shrinkology type you are most likely to be. This is the bit you've been waiting for!

We have combined the well-established research and principles of psychology with a deft bit of insight and analysis to create six distinct 'overeating' categories. The vast majority of people who struggle with their weight will fit one of these. Finding the Shrinkology type which fits you most closely right now is a crucial step in developing your personalised Shrinkology plan. Your approach and attitude to food is, of course, completely unique to you and based on your very own suite of influences, susceptibilities, strengths and weaknesses. But we have found distinctions which help us clearly define each type and cherry pick the best hacks and tips to guide your approach to change. The advice you'll find in your Shrinkology type chapter is very specifically designed to hold greatest appeal to you and ultimately to be most effective in getting your head in the best possible place to find and remain at a happy, healthy weight for you.

First and foremost, you should try and answer the questions in the quiz as instinctively as possible. Don't think, just do. You can run through this quiz with family and friends, but do bear in mind that it is designed as a diagnostic tool for adults who struggle with their weight. The algorithms are not suitable or appropriate for children, and the quiz is not designed for idle curiosity so it cannot offer accurate analysis if you are, in fact, happy with your weight.

Your Results

If you are unsure about your Shrinkology diagnosis, ask your partner or a trusted friend to answer the quiz on your behalf – their response might be intriguing and highlight some aspects of your eating behaviour that you're unaware of. Just make sure they are aware of the purpose of Shrinkology and are there to support, not critique your journey. But anyone who is willing to admit they have certain issues with food, and might be occasionally frustrated by repeated failed dieting attempts, should find themselves clearly falling into one of the six Shrinkology categories. You might find you straddle two or even three types and, as we explain in Part Four, your Shrinkology type can change as you move through life.

Second Place

Do make a note of your second highest score as this could indicate influential factors which will also have a bearing on your future weight-maintenance success. You can think of this as your 'rising type' just as keen astrologers pinpoint their 'sun sign' (from their birth date) but also pay attention to influences of their 'rising sign' (which is usually different, and calculated according to the actual time of birth). It is certainly worth reading through both chapters as any duality in Shrinkology type might explain conflicting traits worth addressing. By tailoring your approach and personalising your plan, you stand a much better chance of success.

ARE YOU A . . .

Rebel who's either fully
immersed in a diet or
thoroughly 'off message'

Gourmet who lives to
entertain and indulge

Scrambler forever nibbling,
grazing, snacking on the hoof

Soother who finds comfort
and solace in food

Traditional adhering to
deeply established dietary
conventions

Magpie flitting from one
sparkly new diet plan to
another?

TAKE THE QUIZ TO FIND OUT.

Which of these most closely describes your friendship style?

A My friends are *extremely* important to me, but I struggle to keep up

B I enjoy the company of people who share my interests

C I have a small number of very core 'best' friends

D My partner/family are my best friends

E I'm not too interested in making new friends, I stick close to my old buddies

F I enjoy meeting new people and building new friendships

What is your most-cherished dream?

A To live a fabulous life free from mundanity

B To achieve tip-top health

C To be truly, deeply happy

D To be mortgage- and debt-free and financially secure

E To be the best of the best in everything I do

F To get to the end of each day without some mini disaster

If you invite friends over for dinner you are most likely to serve up:

A Fine food made from exquisite ingredients, laboriously prepared and beautifully presented

B A healthy and nutritious meal featuring the latest superfood ingredients

C A simple but delicious curry with rice, naan and all the trimmings

D Shepherd's pie with peas/carrots or lasagne (with garlic bread)

E Steaks (preferably medium rare)

F Pre-prepared chicken/salmon breasts with bagged salad

When someone says CAKE do you think:

A 'Which recipe is this? What are the ingredients?'

B 'Does it contain gluten? Sugar? Refined flour? Is it organic?'

C 'Mmmm, delicious!'

D 'If only I had a cup of tea to go with it'

E 'No thanks, I'm trying to be good …oh go on then'

F 'Can you wrap me a slice to go?'

How would you best describe your grocery shopping style?

A I like to browse independent delis and shop locally when possible

B I'm a fan of health food shops and the 'free from' aisles

C I find it hard to stick to my list and I'm easily tempted by offers

D I stick closely to my usual shopping list or my online 'favourites'

E I'll grab something at the express supermarket close to work

F I have an online food delivery every week and I'm always on the look-out for BOGOF deals

Which celebrity impresses you most?

A Barack Obama

B Gwyneth Paltrow

C Oprah Winfrey

D David Attenborough

E Bear Grylls

F Davina McCall

What kind of books do you prefer?

A World events/politics

B Literary prize winners

C Romance

D Celebrity autobiographies

E Personal development/specialist magazines

F Audio books

What movie genre is your favourite?

A A foreign film with subtitles

B True stories/docu-dramas

C Romantic comedies

D Classic action movies like James Bond

E Horror

F Sci-fi

What's your preferred breakfast option?

A Homemade muffin warm from the oven or organic Greek yoghurt
B Green juice or smoothie
C Porridge
D Cornflakes or toast and jam/marmalade
E Protein shake
F Black coffee

Your perfect holiday would be:

A The latest word in high-end luxury
B A fastidiously researched city break with a packed itinerary
C A super-chilled villa/beach/pool holiday
D The same place you love to go back to each year
E High-octane adventure/trekking
F Fun family holidays that involve inevitable compromise

What's your perfect kind of car?

A Lexus (high-end luxury)
B Tesla (economical/environmentally sound)
C Volvo (super-safe)
D Land Rover 4x4 (practical/useful in all conditions)
E Porsche (sexy sports car)
F Ford S-Max (practical/useful)

What's your confrontational style?

A What confrontation? I'm usually right
B I try to read the signs before working out the best option
C I'll usually do anything necessary to find a swift resolution even
   if this means compromise
D I try to avoid conflict and keep things to myself if I can
E I've been known to flounce off in a huff
F I'm good at conflict resolution and sorting things out

What's your preferred snack option?

A Smoked almonds or olives

B Granola bar

C Chocolate

D Biscuits

E Energy ball

F Diet cola

What would you typically choose for lunch on the hop?

A Homemade soup with sourdough bread and cold French butter

B A packaged salad

C A baked potato with cheese and baked beans

D Ham or cheese sandwich on sliced bread (pre-packed)

E Canteen meal or pub lunch

F Chocolate or a couple of biscuits

Chocolate of choice?

A Minimum 85% cocoa solids

B Cacao nibs

C Quality Street/Celebrations

D Cadbury's Dairy Milk

E Chilli-infused chocolate

F Freddo, Finger of Fudge, fun-sized Milky Way

How do you best like to chill in your spare time?

A With friends, food and wine

B Reading or researching

C Box set/Netflix

D DIY/gardening

E Working towards my latest goal/challenge

F What spare time?

What's your preferred work style?

A Entrepreneurial: I like to forge ahead and find new opportunities

B Flexible: I'm happy to balance work from home with the office

C Collaborative: I strive to ensure the team is happy and effective

D Conventional: I like a clear plan and set deadlines

E Managerial: I'm happiest when others let me take charge

F Eclectic/diverse: Some of my best work is done at night

What is your favourite tipple?

A Pastis/schnapps/brandy

B Obscure label gin

C Prosecco

D Whisky/Rioja

E Beer

F White wine (in a large glass)

What is your favourite drink on the go?

A Fresh ground coffee

B Smoothie

C Latte with a flavoured syrup

D Tea

E Energy drink

F Instant coffee

What do you look for in food labels?

A I prefer to buy fresh artisan food which doesn't have labels

B I scrutinise the labels looking for sugar derivatives, preservatives and gluten

C I rarely look at food labels

D I'm brand loyal for familiar names from my childhood (Heinz, Kraft, etc.)
and I don't tend to look at nutritional information.

E I'll check protein content

F I'm more interested in price, offers and deals

RESULTS

Mostly As: You could be a GOURMET

You love food – but not just any food. It has to be the finest you can find. The process of sourcing and preparing food is as important to you as the ingredients, and hosting well-catered parties is a outlet for your exuberant personality. You have a flair for storytelling and you are socially adept. Your curiosity and fascination also spans current affairs, politics, and you have a deep interest in those around you. Any negative issues with food and eating behaviour only appear because you find it incomprehensible not to consume the best food and drink – surely that's what life is all about?

Mostly Bs: You could be a MAGPIE

Magpies love to experiment with sparkly new health approaches. You are a trendsetter in many things, moving on from the 'next big thing' before most of your friends have even heard of it. Your keen investigative skills spill over to all areas of life – you are the go-to person to organise holidays and you are flawless in planning and execution. You also keep an eye on all health news and file it away in your vast memory. The Magpie can quickly lose interest in one diet plan and switch to the next, causing confusion (and overeating), as well as diet fatigue.

Mostly Cs: You could be a SOOTHER

Soothers are highly intuitive, and you care deeply for those around you. You soak up other's pain and heartache and, as a truly compassionate soul, you strive to make everyone happy. Food is truly comforting due to its neurochemical and rewarding effects that you don't receive elsewhere, so you seek to self-soothe with food. This makes it very hard to resist carb-laden foods and stick to diets when feelings start to peek out from under the surface.

Mostly Ds: You could be a TRADITIONAL

As a Traditional, you hold your core values very dear. You have great respect for law and authority and you strive to 'do the right thing'. You know what you like and what you don't and you're not comfortable taking risks. You do like the idea of adventure and spontaneity, but it takes quite a bit of persuading. Friendships and relationships might take longer to build, but once established they are secure. The Traditional sticks close to long-established patterns of eating and will be frustrated by changes in nutritional dogma and the fact that the old dietary rules and portion sizes no longer serve to keep you slim.

Mostly Es: You could be a REBEL

The Rebel is a very black and white thinker – success and goal-meeting are extremely important. You take everything to the max and you're more than happy to lead by example. You're no shirker, and you will exercise to the point of exhaustion, but you'll think nothing of meeting friends in a bar afterwards and drinking double the calories you just burned in the gym. You'll show exemplary willpower and stick to the toughest, most rigid diet plan – with impressive results – then blow everything on an all-you-can-eat buffet.

Mostly Fs: You could be a SCRAMBLER

The Scrambler is busy. Really busy. Whether you're juggling young children, ageing parents, a demanding job, committee work, voluntary positions, you love the challenge of keeping all those plates spinning. For you, life would feel dull if every minute wasn't a multi-tasking challenge. But amid all this organised chaos, it is all too easy to forget to take care of yourself – it can be tough to work out which plate you are going to have to drop to make room. With so little time for proper meals you graze and nibble your way through the day or find yourself starving and out of control in the evenings.

Chapter 6
Shrinkology Fundamentals

Your Shrinkology Fundamentals are the common sense rules and the basic foundations for a healthy relationship with food, regardless of your type. This section is to chaotic eating what sleep hygiene is to insomnia, it is your first step to becoming truly Shrinktastic and regaining control over what, when and how you eat.

The impulsive among you will have already turned to your type chapter and you might just be drifting back here as an afterthought. We strongly urge you, whatever your type, to start here. This is the place to get a good robust underpinning before you layer up with your individual Shrinkology tips. If you really want to find and stick to a happy, healthy weight *long term*, this chapter is the essential first step.

Your Shrinktastic Home

No matter how frenetic your lifestyle, home forms the true heart of your Shrinkology plan. Whether you spend the bulk of your time in the kitchen, you idle away hours in front of the TV in the living room or you only nip back for a few hours each night to use the bathroom and bed, it is very important that the place you call home is set up to maximise the effectiveness and success of your Shrinkology journey.

Your Shrinktastic kitchen

Give yourself the best possible chance of success by transforming your kitchen from a place of temptation to one of health and nutrition.

- Clear work surfaces of tempting treats – the more time you spend at home, and in the kitchen, the more important it is to hide the 'tempting' food.
- Place a full fruit bowl within easy reach (and keep it topped up, fresh and attractive) – studies show consumption of fruit increases if it is accessible and appealing.

FOOD ON DISPLAY

Research by professor Brian Wansink of New York's Cornell University shows tempting foods on display in the kitchen correlates strongly with weight gain.[71] He found his researchers could roughly predict a person's excess weight by the food they have sitting out on the kitchen work top:

Fizzy drinks on display – add 13kg (29lb) in weight
Diet drinks – add 11kg (24lb)
Breakfast cereal – add 9.5 (21lb)
Crisps/tortilla chips – add 3.5 (8lb)
Biscuits – add 4kg (9lb)
Fruit – subtract 3kg (7lb)

- Banish unhealthy processed food, regardless of who eats it. It is good parenting (and *not* cruel) to empty the 'treat drawer'. At the very least, make it smaller and inaccessible (to you as well as them).

- Don't think of unhealthy food like this as 'banned', because banning anything makes it immeasurably more appealing. Understand that if you don't have biscuits, chocolate, ice cream or crisps in the house, you are dramatically reducing your opportunities to eat them. The same rule applies to alcohol. Don't have it in the house and don't drink at home (unless you're entertaining).

- Bring healthy cooking ingredients to the front of cupboards and arrange prominently within reach (you are three times more likely to eat the first food you see in the cupboard than the fifth one). Move any remaining tempting treats to the back of kitchen cabinets.[68] In the absence of doughnuts, even a waxy bar of cooking chocolate can seem super-appealing!

- Wrap tempting foods (like cake or leftover pizza) in foil and stash them in the salad drawer, then move fruit and vegetables to an eye-level shelf. You'll be so much more successful if you see healthy options when you peer into the fridge.

- Wash and cut up carrots, celery, cucumber and cherry tomatoes and display in clear-sided containers to catch the eye when the snacking demons open the fridge door. Or add pre-cut vegetables to your essentials shopping list.

- Use coloured plates for every day and keep white crockery for entertaining. Studies show food appears to be more appealing and delicious when displayed on a white plate, and we eat more slowly off dishes that contrast with the colour of our food.[69]

- Shrink your plates. Studies also show using 25cm (10 inch) or even 23cm (9 inch) plates and 450ml (16oz) bowls could cut food consumption by 22 per cent. Never use very large bowls (e.g. 4 litre/7 pint capacity) as this can increase food intake by over 50 per cent.[70]

- Don't forget the cutlery. You can reduce the amount you eat by a further 14 per cent simply by using a tablespoon to serve yourself rather than a ladle or tongs.

- When feeding family and friends, 'plate up' (i.e. subtly police and enforce healthy portion control) before serving people their food, as research shows we eat whatever is on our plate and, without thinking, can easily consume 30 per cent more calories when given larger portions. But feel free to generously place extra salad and vegetables as a free-for-all on the table.[71]

Your Shrinktastic living space

You can make where you tend to relax on the sofa at the end of a hard day more Shrinktastic with a few subtle changes to limit or restrict any unknown traps and healthy eating hurdles:

- Take a look at your furniture layout. Is everything arranged for maximum TV viewing convenience? Consider re-arranging the furniture subtly to favour socialising and conversation rather than TV viewing. Watching TV uses less cognitive capacity than interacting with others, so our minds will still seek out food when slumped in front of the telly, leading to mindless grazing.[72]
- Set a house rule of one screen only in the living room to encourage communication, preventing the mind from drifting to unwanted thoughts about food.
- Whilst you re-arranging the furniture, have a think. Is there room for an exercise bike/stepper/weights in front of the TV? They might not match your carefully co-ordinated cushion covers, but if you're mostly sedentary, they could save your life. Just sitting on the bike with your legs free-wheeling for an hour while you watch TV is better than sitting alone. But better still, ramp it up a little during the ad breaks to get your heart rate really lifted.
- Ban the evening snacking habit. We can easily notch up hundreds of calories by mindlessly nibbling peanuts, crisps or biscuits in front of the TV. This can be very difficult to stop, so you might find it easier to cut back by making snacking slightly boring,

time-consuming or less convenient. Try telling yourself you can snack, but only when standing, or only if the TV is off, or you're not on your phone, or only if you've eaten a piece of fruit first.

• Keep a full glass of water within arm's reach, but anything else (such as snacks) on a table 2m (6ft) away so you have to get out of your chair to reach them.

• Keep wrappers, cans and bottles within view until the end of the evening as a subtle visual reminder of what you're consuming. It might just nudge you to stopping earlier or sooner than you would if the surfaces were regularly cleared.

Become a Shrinktastic sleeper

If you aren't getting quite enough good-quality sleep every night, you are going to find it much more difficult to reach and stick to a healthy weight, so taking steps to maximise good sleep is an important Shrinkology Fundamental.

Tiredness boosts appetite, making you more vulnerable to cravings, and more likely to abandon your healthy eating intentions and eat fatty and sugary foods as your fatigued brain searches for energy to keep it going. One study showed just five days on four hours' sleep a night (when you're used to seven or eight hours) could result in consuming 296 more calories the following day.[73]

About a third of the general population experience insomnia,[74] with many more of us having the odd bad night now and again. Brain imaging shows that there is increased brain activity in areas associated with food-related reward after a lack of sleep, inferring that those with poor sleep have a heightened awareness of food around them.[75] Poor sleep primes you to seek out high-calorie food because the tired brain knows that food equals calories and calories equal energy, which is what your body and brain desperately need.

One night of disturbed or fragmented sleep can make you hungrier than normal because the glucagon-like peptide (GLP-1), which lets the brain know it's full, is reduced after fractured sleep.[76] This can also lead to afternoon snacking, as concentrations of insulin spike later in the day in response to this disruption. Weight gain can also contribute to sleep problems which can lead to a vicious cycle whereby you don't sleep so you're hungry, but additional pounds cause breathing issues such as snoring and sleep apnoea, resulting in rubbish sleep and so on …

So what's the Shrinkology Sleep Solution? Simple: aim to get 7–8 hours of good-quality sleep every night if you can. There's nothing big or clever about cutting back on this free and delicious lifeline.

- Dial down the 'noise'. If you are prone to insomnia, make a conscious effort to avoid any food and drink, stimulating activities or worries or concerns which might be keeping your body and mind active after bedtime.
- Try and move around for at least 30 minutes a day, even if you are feeling exhausted . Avoid scheduling this 3–4 hours before bedtime, as intense exercise can activate the body and mind.
- Try not to eat 2 hours before bed. Heavy and calorie-laden meals might initially make you feel drowsy, but eating late in the evening will challenge the digestive system and potentially disrupt sleep. Spicy foods can make it hard to fall asleep and stay asleep, too.
- Don't go to bed really hungry, as this can trigger the release of the stress hormone cortisol, which might wake you up in the early hours. Ensure your evening meal contains protein, healthy fats and slow release carbohydrates to see you through to breakfast.
- Cut back on caffeine. You might think coffee and tea don't bother you, and everyone feels the effects of caffeine differently, but if you're not getting good restorative sleep every night, it is certainly worth cutting back – or at the very least, avoiding coffee and tea in the afternoon and evening. Be warned, de-caffeinated drinks are only partially de-caffeinated – not fully un-caffeinated so, if you're

sensitive, you could still be receiving a stimulating effect. NB Chocolate contains caffeine too!

- Avoid smoking (or vaping) within 4 hours of going to bed. Nicotine is a stimulant, too.
- Watch the booze! It's a common misconception that a nightcap aids sleep, and although a few drinks might make us feel drowsy (they act as a sedative, effectively knocking us out), alcohol disrupts our ability to enter the deeply restorative stages of sleep. Every measure of alcohol consumed (even during the day) could equate to an hour's loss of sleep.

SET A BEDTIME ROUTINE

Establishing a regular and familiar bedtime routine to help establish a strong link in our brain with sleep:

- set an immovable bedtime (7–8 hours before your regular wake-up time);
- start winding down an hour before bed, switching off the TV, computer and putting your phone away;
- instead switch to reading or listening to music;
- have a cup of hot milk or herbal tea;
- take a warm shower or bath (this brings body temperature up just before bed, ensuring that core temperature drops when you get into bed, so signalling sleep).

Your Shrinktastic bedroom

It's not just how we sleep, but where we sleep too. There are many tweaks that can be carried out to make your bedroom more sleep-friendly.

- **Use noise blockers.** If you are a light sleeper, easily disturbed by sudden noises or from other people in the house, the hum of white noise from an electric fan can help de-sensitise an over-vigilant brain. This continuous sound blocks out disrupting noises that jar us from slumber. Keep disposable foam ear plugs by your bed to pop in on those nights when you are infuriatingly alert.
- **Block out the light.** Try turning off all the lights and holding your hand in front of your face. If you can see your hand, it's still too light and this could be disrupting your sleep. If blackout blinds or heavy curtains aren't an option, a simple soft eye mask can do the trick.

SLEEPING AWAY FROM HOME

If you find you sleep badly when you're away from home, consider taking a pillowcase with you. Often your brain will switch to natural survival mode for the first night in a new place, unwittingly scanning for potential danger. But if you lie your head on something that smells reassuringly of your own familiar detergent, it can reassure an over-active mind.

- **Be cool.** Aim to have your bedroom at a steady 18°C through the night.
- **Banish all electronic equipment from the bedroom.** This includes your smartphone. Even very small amounts of blue light from the screen have been shown to disrupt sleep patterns, and any buzzing or beeping will unsettle your sleep even if you're not consciously aware of the noise during the night.
- **Invest in a simple alarm clock.** A light clock is a lovely idea – using light to gently wake you in the morning, rather than a juddering noise, but turn it to face the wall so you are not tempted to check

the time if you wake up in the night and then unwittingly torture yourself with recriminations about how little sleep you're getting or how soon it is until morning.

CHANGING BAD HABITS FOR GOOD ONES

The best way to ditch a stubborn bad habit is to replace it with a better one. Buy exotic herbal tea bags and use that 'ah the kids are finally in bed, it's me time now' feeling as a cue to boil the kettle rather than reach for the wine. Ask for olives instead of bread when you're out for a meal. Ditch your scrolling-through-your-phone-in-bed habit and start that book you've been meaning to read for ages.

But be warned – to make the change stick, a new habit must be repeated until it's as strong as the old habit, which may be a lot of times if the old habit is deeply ingrained. Repetition is key. Studies show it can take 18–254 days (with an average of 66 days) for a new habit to stick.

Careful planning can help. As a cue, choose something that happens every day, such as brushing your teeth, walking to work or eating lunch. To bridge the gap between the cue and the behaviour in the early stages of habit formation, try using a visual reminder, like leaving walking shoes on the car's passenger seat or posting a note on the mirror for a habit triggered by tooth-brushing.

Your Shrinktastic bathroom

For many people who struggle with their weight, the bathroom can be a source of stress. If unflattering lighting makes you unhappy when you look in the mirror, consider dimmer switches or softer, more flattering bulbs. Position mirrors so you don't inadvertently catch sight of your reflection when stepping in and out of the shower. Instead you can ramp up the self-love a little by turning your bathroom into your own home spa with super-soft towels and deliciously relaxing or invigorating products. Try instilling a family rule that bathroom time is everyone's individual 'me' time, which can only be disturbed in emergencies.

Your bathroom is also the mostly likely home of your weighing scales. Debate rages as to whether and how often we should jump on the scales. Certainly there are plenty of successfully slim people who *never* weigh themselves, and others who swear by a weekly weigh-in. Some people keep tabs on their body size via their clothes (a too-tight waistband signalling time for action), and others jump on the scales every morning.

It is important to be aware that scales can be fickle and your weight can fluctuate by as much as 1kg (2lb) in any given day, but the most compelling research evidence seems to point at the importance of keeping a close watch on your weight.

Weigh yourself every day if you like, but certainly once a week, even when you reach your happy healthy weight. It is so much easier to bring any newfound behaviours or dietary slips back into line when you've only got a couple of pounds to lose.

One study found dieters who weigh themselves daily lose the most weight – the average period between weight checks without gaining weight was 5.8 days. It seems the longer you wait between weigh-ins, the more weight you are likely to gain. Women who weighed themselves nearly every day over the course of the year not only lost more weight than those who kept infrequent tabs on their number, but they also maintained their weight loss.[77]

If you haven't weighed yourself for years, be brave. Try not to be frightened about what you see on the scales. The numbers are arbitrary, but the differential is important. If you want to lose weight it can be hugely motivating to see the numbers fall – and if you haven't weighed yourself at your heaviest, what incentive do you have? How can you celebrate your great Shrinkology success?

It is worth considering scales that also measure fat percentage, as this is another factor which can keep you motivated if emotional eating starts to get out of control.

Most be sensible about what you consider to be your 'ideal' weight. Everything changes as we get older and it is healthier to aim to your 'true' weight rather than some random weight you rather liked yourself at when you were in your teens or early twenties. Your Shrinkology weight (see opposite) should be a good indication of a realistic, achievable weight to aim for.

How To Find Your Shrinkology Weight

1. How much did you weigh when you were 18 years old (without dieting?) in lbs or kg (e.g. 70 kg, 11 stone, 154lb)
2. How much did you weigh at your heaviest (not including pregnancy weight) (e.g. 77kg, 12 stone, or 168lb)
3. How much did you weigh at your lightest after the age of 18, with or without having dieted? (e.g.64kg, 10 stone, or 140lb)
4. What is your current weight? (e.g.77kg, 12 stone, or 168lb)

Add together your answers to questions 1 and 2 (154 + 168 = 322) and divide by 2 (161). The result is A.

Add together your answers to questions 3 and 4 (140 + 168 = 308) and divide by 2 (154). The result is B.

Now add A and B (161 + 154 = 315) and divide by 2 (157 or 11 stone 2lb).

This final number is a good achievable target weight.

Your Shrinkology house

There are fundamental changes you can make to your environment to boost your chances of Shrinkology success. If you only do one thing in each room, these tricks will make a huge difference:

Bedroom
Place eye mask and ear plugs on bedside table to ensure complete dark and silence for a good night's sleep

Bathroom
Get a good set of scales to weigh yourself every week

Garage
Stash tempting foods in an inconvenient place so although it's not out of bounds it is out of reach

Living/Sitting Room
Make room for an exercise bike/stepper/weights positioned in front of TV for max opportunistic activity

Kitchen
Clear kitchen work surfaces to reduce your unconscious exposure (and eating without realising what you are doing) and put a full fruit bowl on display

Shrinktastic food shopping

Supermarkets are cleverly designed and laid out to tempt you to buy more, to try foods you might not have tried before, and to pick up the packaged processed foods with the highest profit margin. That's why it's so easy to pop in for one or two things and find yourself unloading a complete trolley full on to the conveyor belt.

Shopping when you're hungry is a bad strategy as people tend to toss higher-calorie food into their trolley, even if they're not actually buying more items of food.[78] But if nipping to the shops on your way home is the only option, try chewing gum as you move around the store – minty freshness in your mouth can help short-circuit cravings, making it harder for your brain to imagine the sensory details of crunchy crisps or creamy ice cream.

The key to Shrinktastic food shopping is to be on your guard, and be prepared. A successful bit of food shopping is fundamental to your Shrinkology success because food that's bought here gets brought home, and food at home gets eaten.

- Stop buying unhealthy food. Make a pact with yourself, and write a shopping list of good, healthy foods you enjoy eating and plan to stick to that list and aim not to waver.
- Divide and conquer. Use your jacket or a newspaper to divide the trolley in half as a visual aid to ensure 50 percent of your food shopping is healthy salads, vegetables and fruit.[79]
- Spend plenty of time browsing the fresh fruit and vegetable aisles. This is the best place to be, so investigate unfamiliar fruit and vegetables to broaden your horizons and don't rush this bit.
- Have a plan. Next, head straight to the fresh meat/dairy or produce sections, or the aisle with canned and frozen fruit and vegetables while your shopping enthusiasm is still high, and before you the hit processed food hell of those brightly coloured central aisles.

- Be mindful. Each time you put something in your trolley, ask yourself, 'is this going to help me achieve my ideal size and weight?'
- Ban the booze. Wipe alcohol off your usual shopping list.
- Pat yourself on the back. Acknowledge your good food choices. This provides reassurance and affirmation to seal the neural pathways you have created, making these new behaviours more likely to stick.

SHRINKTASTIC ONLINE SHOPPING

If you're the sort to be tempted by offers and distracted by the sights and smells of the supermarket, you might find that switching to online shopping is a great way to stick to your healthy guns – and it could save you enough time in your busy schedule to squeeze in an exercise session or at the very least to create a vegetable-packed home-cooked meal.

- Create a shopping list of healthy essentials and aim not to stray.
- Invest a little time upfront to work out the healthy basics you regularly use each week plus interesting extras which might crop up in recipes you'd like to try.
- Aim to add a new, unfamiliar item of fruit or vegetable (that includes pulses) to your list each week.
- Remove the unhealthy extras which might have crept on to your 'favourites' list to ensure every item on the list is fundamentally healthy and any off-piste additions are new (and thoughtfully considered) ones.

Shrinktastic at work

The workplace can be fraught with toxic eating triggers – from the tea trolley to the office feeder. To keep your workplace shrinkology-approved, keep cakes and sweets off your desk. Studies show people who keep a bowl of sweets within reach at work tend to believe they're more difficult to resist and eat more than if the sweets were tucked away. Just keeping sweets in opaque, rather than clear containers helps curb cravings, too.[80]

Become great at saying 'No'. It can be very hard to turn down that 'special' slice of birthday cake. But you can strengthen your 'just say no' muscle even with the most demanding friends and colleagues by practising your 'no' script at home. Practise stating out loud what you're trying to achieve: 'I want to develop a better relationship with food, lose some weight and keep it off, so no thank you as the cake isn't part of this goal.' You don't need to say this when cake is proffered, but it is very useful to have this as back up in your mind. So, when the cake comes out, try this:

1. Be very clear in your mind that you don't want the cake, otherwise the indecisiveness will come across.

2. Say 'no thank you' and if you like, give a version of your rehearsed reason – with conviction!

3. Don't apologise for your choices. Remember you are taking positive steps for you and your future.

4. Brace yourself for the kick-back ('come on, it's only a bit of cake!') and hold your ground.

5. Suggest some other means of celebration, such as: 'Even though I'm not going to have a slice, I'm still here with you celebrating, and that's the important thing.'

Over time, your colleagues will see your determination and will respect you for not bending to pressure.

Your Shrinktastic car

Consuming food outside the home can put us at risk of unconscious overeating and self-sabotage on the dieting front. Shrinkology-proofing your mode of transport can help break poor eating habits.

- Download an audiobook or podcast. This can ease the sort of boredom that might trigger eating if you're the sort to spend long periods of time in the car.
- Have chewing gum on hand. Studies show chewing gum can boost metabolism a little and help weight loss.[81]
- Keep a pack of almonds in the glove compartment for hunger emergencies. Plain unsalted nuts are much harder to overeat than salted, smoked or honey-roasted.
- Instil a 'buy nothing but fuel at filling stations' policy.

The Shrinktastic guide to eating out

Don't let your well-meaning efforts to eat more healthily and achieve a healthy long-term weight spoil your fun. It is important to let your hair down occasionally, eat out, try new foods, indulge and enjoy – life is short, food is delicious and you're worth it! Most restaurants are not a dieter's friend but you can still have fun without having to resort to side salad and water.

- Plan ahead. Decide on an eating strategy before you go in. Check the menu online and decide what you plan to order.
- Take it slowly. Make a point of connecting with the people you are with and slowly savour the taste of your food. Put your fork down after each bite, eating with your non-dominant hand, or take a long, slow deep breath between bites to slow your eating.

WISE UP

Look out for menu tricks which could hold a clue to unhealthy food choices: opting for a food item described as 'buttery' could mean you will be adding an average of 102 calories; anything described as 'crispy' could mean adding 131 more calories; but studies show 'seasoned', 'roasted' or 'marinated' items tend to have 60 fewer calories than their unseasoned, unroasted, or unmarinated counterparts.

- Sit by a window. Studies show people who sit by the window, or in a well-lit part of the restaurant tend to order healthier foods – more salads and fewer desserts – particularly if they sit at high-top bar tables rather than a cosy dark corner.[82] This could be because the visibility makes you subconsciously aware of other people watching you eat – or even that it allows you to see more clearly what's on your plate. It's also worth sitting away from the bar (watching other drinkers 'normalises' drinking, making it easier to order more), and out of sight of a TV screen (distracting).
- Become a menu cynic. Restaurants employ professional 'menu engineers' who show restaurants how to design their menus to guide our eyes to the most profitable items. We tend to read menus in a Z-shaped pattern, starting at the top left, moving to the top right, swinging down through the middle to the bottom left and ending at the bottom right. After an initial sweep, we will check out whatever catches our eye – boxes, bold type, pictures, logos or icons.

BE THE BOSS OF THE BUFFET

An all-you-can-eat buffet is a potential disaster zone for anyone trying to maintain a healthy weight – all that choice laid out before you can be bamboozling for the inveterate dieter. That groaning spread of tempting foods is not just an opportunity to overeat, it carries the potential to break your hard-fought resolve, shatter your plans and throw you into complete diet disarray.

Experts might say there's only one way to not overeat at a buffet – avoid it – but with a little bit of cunning insider information, you can learn to cruise the buffet table, enjoy the food and come away unscathed.

You can counteract any unhealthy eating habits and work a buffet well by trying these tips:
- 'scout' out the buffet before picking up a plate, mentally selecting the healthiest foods and those that fit your eating plan;[83]
- pick up a small plate and cherry pick your favourite foods only – fill half your plate with salad or vegetables;[84]
- find a table far away from the buffet and sit with your back to the food;
- eat slowly, chewing each mouthful 15 times;
- wait 20 minutes, and don't return to the buffet unless you are still hungry.

Get moving!

The health benefits of regular exercise are now unequivocal, and getting active is a very important part of any personalised Shrinkology plan. For a start, being a little active every day is enough to reduce your risk of stroke, type 2 diabetes, depression, Alzheimer's and even some cancers. It can elevate your mood, make you feel good about yourself, alleviate anxiety and help with stress management. It can also improve sleep, protect you against osteoporosis, provide rewarding new skills and challenges and – if you pick the right kind of activity for you – it really can add fun to your life.

But, very importantly for the Shrinkology message, there's absolutely no doubt that combining exercise with a healthy diet is a more effective way to lose and maintain weight than just cutting back on food alone. Certainly numerous studies show weight-loss programmes which combine diet and physical activity are more successful than those that don't. One reason is the calorie burn – important if you're going to be able to create the calorie deficit that is key to weight loss. But exercise also builds muscles which increases your resting calorie burn and raises your metabolism even when you're sitting around doing nothing. That's because muscle is metabolically active which means that it requires fuel in the form of calories just to keep things ticking over. For instance, just 500g (1lb) of muscle burns 75 calories a day, but 500g (1lb) of fat burns just 8 calories a day. The more muscle you have the more calories you consume and, if you don't overeat, the more fat you will burn.

The good news is you don't have to become an exercise freak to be Shrinktastic. Research has shown that a brisk walk four times a week is enough to reduce body fat and improve the way your body metabolises food.[85] But the more activity you can build into your daily life the better.

The ideal exercise prescription combines cardiovascular exercise (getting you out of breath) plus resistance training (with weights, bands or using your body weight) to build muscles and keep you strong. It's worth the effort because if you work hard enough to replace 10lb of fat with 10lb of muscle, your body will burn roughly 40 more calories a day at rest. This doesn't sound like much, but it swiftly accumulates to become 280 extra calories burned a week, and 1,120 a month – that's enough to lose weight without restricting your food intake at all!

So, if you can, add a few press-ups, squats and lunges to your fitness programme, or try an exercise DVD that incorporates resistance bands or weights (whether that's using bottles of water or dumb-bells), or alternate your aerobics class with a weight-training one.

Getting off the starting blocks

If you loathed PE at school and you've spent a lifetime avoiding Lycra and sweat, happily watching sport from the comfort of your sofa instead, it can be difficult to know where to start becoming active. You'll find clever personalised exercise recommendations in each type chapter, so once you've found one that sounds promising, aim to start slowly.

At first, if you're new to exercise, just aim to be active – even for just a few minutes – every single day, and vary what you do. Set small goals (a 10-minute walk, 15 minutes of slow pedalling on an exercise bike, gentle swimming) and stick with it. The first step, and a strong Shrinkology Fundamental, is to make a pact with yourself. No shirking. *Make* time for activity and exercise, don't try to *find* time. Put it in your diary and, if you are physically able, do something active every single day. Forever.

Even if clearing a diary spot is difficult, every morning, just ask yourself: 'What kind of activity am I going to do today?' Or better still, set your intention and block out a section of time in your diary the night before. Your fitness will improve swiftly, so as soon as an activity feels easy, increase the length of time and intensity. Aim to raise your heart rate to the point where you can still talk, but you are too puffed to sing the words to a song, and stay there for progressively longer periods of time each day.

When you have reached a good basic level of fitness (you can happily walk for 30 minutes at a brisk pace) you should feel strong enough to investigate classes and clubs in your area and to start making exercise a long-term habit that sticks. It is important to inject as much variety as possible into your exercise regime because muscles are highly adaptable (and boredom thresholds are low). If you don't vary your exercise regime, your muscles will become efficient and burn fewer calories than if you mixed your physical activities. The key is to vary your routine and also to introduce increasingly intense sessions within your exercise programme.

Just aim to do something active and to do it often. Pick an activity you enjoy enough to keep doing, regularly, without having to be reminded. Even if you don't ever quite get to the point where you can honestly say you love exercise, you can at the very least learn to love what exercise can do for you.

Chapter 7
Shrinkology
Food Rules

Whatever your Shrinkology type, circumstances or lifestyle, there are fundamental principles of healthy eating which we urge you to adopt before you consider any diet plan. For some, this could be enough to see long-term weight loss and maintenance at a healthy weight. Others might find they need to embellish these fundamentals with type-specific recommendations (see individual type chapters). But these principles will certainly enhance your health and happiness.

Plan for health

Don't make the mistake of skidding into each week on two wheels with an empty fridge and nothing but porridge oats and a can of baked beans in the cupboards. There's little more likely to get you grabbing a takeaway or pulling something entirely unsuitable out of the muddied depths of your freezer.

Instead, set an alarm on your phone for early Sunday evening and set aside an hour of quiet time on your own to look through your plans for the week, check the fridge and kitchen cupboards, and think about what you're going to eat and when. Can you go shopping? Do a quick online shop? What can you make from the contents of the cupboards? Do you have some emergency homemade soup in the freezer which you could get out in the morning to defrost? Can you get a few things ready to put in the slow cooker before you go to work in the morning?

Eat a little less

If you are unhappy with your weight, the reason could be staring you in the face – you could be eating too much of the wrong foods.

The average daily calorie intake for most people is now around 2,757 calories per day, but the recommended consumption levels (according to the NHS) has for a long time been considerably lower at 2,000 for women and 2,400 for men. There is a compelling new argument that even these levels have been set too high. In 1900 our average daily calorie intake was 2,100 calories. Ok, there was quite a bit of malnutrition around to skew those figures, and plenty of people went hungry, but we were certainly eating less and moving more – most labour was manual and walking was the main mode of transport. Now tough new guidelines from Public Health England are urging us all to cut back to 1800 calories a day (1600 on meals and 200 on snacks).

If you're regularly enjoying more than 2,500 calories a day and you're not particularly active, it's not rocket science to see why weight maintenance might be a bit tricky for you. You might be able to blame creeping weight gain on the fact that we really do need fewer calories as we get older. Eat too many and they'll turn to fat.

It is also important to realise that once you start on your Shrinkology journey, and as you lose weight, your metabolic demands are likely to shrink with your waistline. This means even if you arrive at a happy, healthy weight, you will need to continue to eat fewer calories than you used to eat to stay there. One of the reasons yo-yo dieting is such a common phenomenon is that people frequently arrive at their diet goal, or plateau at a frustratingly immovable place just higher than their goal, then abandon the dietary restrictions, returning to their old eating habits and portion sizes. That's why the weight piles back on.

In the quest for a happy, healthy Shrinktastic weight, you might have to accept progressively eating less as you shrink, then a little experimenting with the amounts you can and can't eat when you get there. If you eat the right foods, you won't feel hungry, but you will learn to slow the acceleration of age-related weight gain.

It might seem like a drastic cut back if you've become accustomed to eating considerably more, but your body and brain will swiftly adapt. Aim to shrink your portions slightly, skip the snacks and (depending on your age and your activity levels) aim keep your total calorie count closer to the level we enjoyed in the 1950s. It is important to ensure the food you do eat is as nutrient-dense as possible. Shun the empty calories of fizzy drinks and sugary treats, and make every mouthful count towards your health and vitality.

TRY THE BROCCOLI TEST

When you next feel the desire to reach for a snack, imagine the snack food is a plate of broccoli. Do you still feel the urge to eat? If you're not sure, try nibbling on a stick of raw broccoli. Are you really hungry?

Let salad or vegetables fill half your plate at every meal if you can. Vegetables are your secret weapon and naturally very low in calories, so by filling at least half your plate with vegetables you will be naturally cutting back and boosting your nutritional input at the same time.

No matter what you thought about vegetables when you were growing up, no matter how picky you might have been, this is a non-negotiable route to long-term health. Trust us – if you can learn to pep up boring veg with olive oil, butter, salt, spices, lemon juice and chilli flakes, you open your doors to a whole new world of life-enhancing deliciousness. Ask for extra vegetables when you're out, eat vegetable snacks and shoehorn vegetables into breakfast if you can (a grilled tomato with your omelette? Spinach or kale in your smoothie?). Aim for maximum variety and a range of colours every time. Don't make the mistake of thinking the '5-a-day' rule is mostly fruit (an orange, an apple, some grapes, fruit juice and a carrot), as you'll be nutritionally better off with four (or eight) portions of vegetables and one piece of fruit.

Eat your fruit, don't drink it

Save the money you used to spend on fruit juice and smoothies and enjoy real fruit instead. There are beneficial plant compounds stored in the pith of oranges and satsumas, great disease fighting nutrients in apple skin and berry pips. This is where you'll get the fibre that helps you feel full and keeps your digestive system motoring and happy.

Nourish your gut bacteria

Earlier on, we explained how unhappy gut bacteria can lead to weight gain and make finding your happy, healthy weight more difficult. Our new understanding of the gut and its microbiome means we're now able to fine-tune our approach to eating to make it even healthier – and even more effective for achieving and attaining a healthy weight. The key to laying the best possible foundations for a healthy gut and a healthy weight is ensuring a diverse population of gut bacteria.

You can support your gut bacteria and make a real difference by trying these tips:

- **CHEW YOUR FOOD WELL** – happy gut bacteria like to feed on food that has been broken down properly.
- **DRINK A LITTLE RED WINE** – it has been shown to improve levels of very beneficial bifida bacteria in the gut.
- **USE APPLE CIDER VINEGAR IN YOUR SALAD DRESSING** – you can buy it from supermarkets) and crunch up crispy seaweed sheets (sold as 'nori sheets' in the sushi section of large supermarkets) into soups and stews.
- **MAKE CLEAR GAPS BETWEEN MEALS AND A LONG NIGHT-TIME FAST** – to give your gut a rest from constantly digesting. This allows the lining of the gut to regenerate and encourages the growth of good bacteria (one type, called Akkermansia, feasts on the mucus that your gut secretes when it is empty – studies show giving this bacteria to overweight mice stopped them becoming obese and developing diabetes altogether[86]).
- **ENJOY GUT-FRIENDLY PREBIOTIC FOODS** (such as onions, garlic, chicory, string beans, wheat bran, celery and tough stems of cabbage or kale) – good microbes love to feast on these. Prebiotics are fibrous foods which are not digested in the small intestine, but continue on down the gut to become an important source of nutrients for the microbiome, promoting the growth of beneficial bacteria.
- **EAT ONE PORTION OF PROBIOTIC YOGHURT, SAUERKRAUT OR KIMCHI EVERY DAY** – this will increase the diversity of your bacteria population by adding new sources in the form of probiotics or 'friendly live bacteria'

Think brown(er)

Switch to wholemeal bread, pasta, rice and flour which contain more nutrients and burn more slowly in your stomach, so keeping you feeling fuller for longer and keeping blood sugar levels steady. And reduce the size of your carbohydrate portions to smaller than you might like: a baked potato shouldn't be bigger than your clenched fist; rather than creating an overflowing bowl with a dollop of sauce on top, put a serving spoon of pasta or rice on the side of your plate, with sauce alongside.

KEY QUESTIONS

At every meal ask yourself: 'What whole grains can I choose? What extra vegetables can I add? Where's my protein? My healthy fats? How colourful is my plate?'

Boost protein

Enjoy meat, fish and eggs, as well as plant protein, in the form of beans and pulses, nuts and seeds, and aim to have some protein with every meal (even breakfast) to keep you feeling fuller for longer. Not only is protein an essential building block for muscle formation (which keeps you strong and burns calories) it also helps activate the release of the satiety hormones which tell us we are full, and stop us eating. Snacks that are high in protein, such as almonds or peanut butter will also trigger the full feeling.

WHAT ABOUT SWEETENERS?

Artificial sweeteners cheat your system into expecting a sugar fix, and in so doing they help maintain your sweet tooth. They can also damage a healthy microbiome (as we showed in Chapter 1).

So best advice might be to use a little sweetener in ever-decreasing quantities (such as Stevia or Xylitol) if it helps to gradually calm your sweet tooth, but aim to nudge sweeteners out of your life too.

Think of desserts as treats

Rein yourself in from any notion that a meal is not complete without a sweet treat. We don't need to finish a meal with sugar, or even fruit. If you eat slowly and deliberately and keep sight of your hunger signalling, you should be happy to walk away from the table without cake or yoghurt. But never say never, as total abstinence is dull and unsustainable unless you're a study-worthy scientific phenomenon. Instead, plan and anticipate those occasions when you know you'll really want a pudding. Feel free to browse the desert menu (if you want to) or if you don't eat out very often, and go ahead and whip up a sumptuous pudding after Sunday lunch with the family. Just make it an occasional, rather than daily, indulgence. Sometimes all you need is a taste, so try a square of good-quality chocolate instead.

Cut back on sugar and processed foods

You can slowly retrain your palette and your gut microbiome by cutting back on sugar, processed and starchy foods. If you focus on feeding the good microbes in your gut a veg-rich healthy diet you will, in time, silence the demands of the sugar-loving ones. Avoid ready meals, takeaways and anything with more than five items on the ingredients list (and words on there your grandmother wouldn't understand). Experiment and cook from scratch as much as you can. Variety is key – don't get stuck in an eating rut.

Healthy fats not low fats

You need fat to feel full. Olive oil, avocados, coconut oil, nuts and seeds release energy more slowly and keep you feeling full for longer. Studies show one tablespoon of full-fat Greek yoghurt is more satisfying than a whole bowl of thin, sweetened low-fat yoghurt.[87] Enjoy the taste, in moderation.

Cutting back on the booze

Whatever your Shrinkology type, one of the most effective steps you can take towards achieving a healthy weight long term is to put a restriction on your intake of alcohol. It is a good move to make for all aspects of your health. Alcohol is high in calories. A regular glass of wine is about 150 cals and a bottle – not tough to get through over the course of a long dinner party evening with friends – will set you back 650 cals. That's equivalent to an extra meal. Take that bottle out of the equation (even only temporarily) and you could be cutting out a whole meal without feeling hungry.

What's more, these days, it can be difficult to know exactly how much we're drinking. A large glass of wine is now equal to a third of a bottle (three glasses with dinner and that's a bottle).When it comes to beers and ciders, a pint may still be a pint but the percentage of alcohol per glass has increased. Beer or lager used to be around 4% alcohol and now it's 4.5–5+%. Those healthy sounding 'low alcohol' beers now on the market were considered to be normal during much of the 20th century. If you've noticed your hangovers getting worse with age, it could be more to do with the generous measures and stronger drinks than your failing ability to 'hold your drink.'

Having a few drinks often impairs your ability to make healthy food choices, both at the time and afterwards. Who craves salad when they've got a crashing hangover? When you're eating out, even one drink is enough to make the bread basket tempting and the fries no longer optional. That's because alcohol affects the frontal lobe of the brain, which is involved with sensible thought and making the right decisions. Studies also show that drinking triggers chemical changes that make the brain primed to find food smells more appealing.[88] One theory is that this could be a sign that your body could be trying to encourage you to eat in order to slow down the speed at which the alcohol is absorbed into the blood.

For some Shrinkology types, complete abstinence works best. Studies show that a month off the booze is enough to drop half a stone without having to make any other changes. It's certainly a great place to start. For other Shrinkology types, cutting back might be more effective. Turn to your chapter for tips and tricks specially designed to suit you and your type, which you can incorporate into your personalised plan.

The Shrinktastic route to effective dieting

For the majority of people, the changes in this chapter will be enough to create the small daily calorie deficit your body needs to return to a healthy and sustainable weight. But if you'd like to kick start a significant period of weight loss, then a proper structured diet plan is also necessary. We are going to give it to you straight here: there is no such thing as the perfect diet. It *is* true that whatever you fancy trying your hand at, you *will* end up consciously reducing your calorie intake and probably lose weight.

However, the statistics show that the vast majority of diets don't work long term. Most dieters will abandon ship and regain the weight they lost. We are not trying to put you off here. Dieting is tough. The key is working out which plans you can maintain in the long term: which plans fit with your lifestyle and personality type.

You'll find low-carb aficionados at every gym, full of the health benefits of ketosis (a state where you body uses fat for fuel). But they will have placed body shape above any desire for cake, biscuits, mashed potato or a glass of Prosecco. There's no such thing as 'low-carb lite'. You're either on the diet, or you're off. It's the same story with meal replacement diets. They might be an effective way to lose weight in the short-term, but long-term, they mean you have to swop a plate of real food for an alternative at least once a day for the rest of your life. Similarly, successful intermittent fasters reach their happy weight, but *still* commit to a 6:1 regime of calorie deficit one day a week to keep it there. The greatest Weight Watcher's success stories are those who stay connected, or run classes themselves.

If you've always struggled with your weight, it's time to be realistic. You can never go back to eating and drinking with the complete abandon that added the extra pounds to start with. The only diets which fit the Shrinkology brief are those which offer a long term plan allowing real food, which you really can incorporate seamlessly and effortlessly into your life, including holidays, parties, weddings ..., and which work for your type.

The Shrinktastic Twist

Yes, there will always be unforeseen dietary swerve balls (the Krispy Kreme gift box, the tempting muffin samples at the coffee shop) but if you have your Shrinkology Fundamentals in place, and your home is Shrinktastic, you will be in a strong and positive place.

Part Three
Shrinkology Types

Now you've got all your healthy eating foundations
in place and you're sure which of the six Shrinkology
Types best describes your emotional and behavioural
approach to food, it's time for the real fun to start!

In your type chapter, you'll find specifically targeted
mind hacks to help ease and mitigate any unhelpful
behaviours, clever type-specific, weight-management
food and exercise tips, and a personalised diet
digest of the weight-loss regimes most likely to
sit comfortably with your personality and lifestyle.
Go ahead and cherry pick the snippets of advice that
resonate most to create your very own, completely
personalised Shrinkology Solution.

Chapter 8
The Gourmet

Who is The Gourmet?

The Gourmet is always ready for fun and radiates energy and enthusiasm. You don't have any problem with living in the moment – you are the moment! Not backwards in coming forwards, you love to get their hands dirty and dive into tasks – you don't need to weigh options up at any great length and you might find you can get a little frustrated with people that spend ('waste') a great deal of time listing pros and cons.

Gourmets are expert storytellers and you are highly adept at keeping your audience on the edge of their seats. The Gourmet feels truly alive when in the company of others – the drama and performance of life are fuel for your passionate personality. Always up to date on current affairs, the Gourmet is as comfortable discussing international politics as they are the latest exquisite food trend. Chores and routine can bore a Gourmet to death – who has time for such things?!? You'd much rather close their eyes and stick a pin in the map than spend 12 months debating where to go next for a holiday. To go somewhere twice, a destination would need to be very special, or perhaps revisited with some first-timers whom you could 'wow' with your insider knowledge.

The Gourmet's house is fantastic – you certainly have a flair for style and you are an open and extremely hospitable person. Guests are made to feel at home and they are free to roam around and lounge in any room. You appreciate the finer things in life and want to share these with others because of your unguarded and sociable nature.

You love eating out, cooking and entertaining – in fact you derive a great sense of worth from social interactions. But you are fiercely loyal and you will keep a close circle of friends very protected and close to your heart.

Everyone wants an invitation to the Gourmet's dinner party. Not only will your food be beyond delicious, but the atmosphere and conversation will be exquisite. No expense will be spared. Your passion for and knowledge of food and drink is encyclopaedic and you love searching out the best-quality ingredients and going off the beaten track to find the perfect deli or wine merchant. Shopkeepers know you well and they look forward to impressing you with their new produce and discussing its provenance at length.

Delicious food is a notable part of your identity. You watch food programmes, collect great cookbooks, follow fellow gourmets on Instagram and shop at specialist delis and fancy supermarkets (because food is just not something that can be skimped on). This doesn't mean you avoid the discount supermarkets: you love exploring, just to nose out fascinating morsels of exotic luxury .

Classic Gourmet eating behaviours

Your love of eating, cooking and entertaining means food is always on your mind, your fridge is packed with delicious delights and your cupboards are heaving with enticing and exotic ingredients – meaning that calorific temptation is always at your fingertips.

- High calorie foods. One look at your food/mood diary is likely to indicate that you're unconsciously consuming far too many calories while cooking, enjoying every delicious mouthful, and quaffing exquisite wine.
- No stop button. You are strident about turning down a food item you dislike, or a meal that is poorly seasoned or of inferior quality, and you don't have any qualms about leaving food on your plate if it doesn't meet your very high expectations. But when you are eating something fantastic, the 'stop when you're full' rules no longer apply.
- Food is your passion, so dinner parties and big restaurant meals will be a regular fixture in your diary – and if you've managed to secure a table at the latest venue, or with the hottest chef, you're going to want to tuck in to the seven-course tasting menu (with a different wine for each course) rather than a lightly dressed salad starter.
- You could be a feeder. With a strong reputation to uphold and an obligation to feed others inside and outside the home, much of your spare time will be occupied with preparing cakes for fund-raisers, or nourishing meals for the children, making yours a very food-oriented existence.
- Restriction is off the menu. You hate the idea of 'low' anything, so everything in your kitchen and everything you pick up outside of it will be full fat and full sugar.
- You find choice hard. You tend to be indecisive when eating out in restaurants, because you can't bear the prospect of being disappointed. This can leave you hankering after everyone else's meals when the food arrives and 'trying' tasters from everyone else. Plus dessert.

Gourmet case study

Lucas hasn't eaten all day – because tasting is definitely not eating. He is hosting his annual house party tonight which consists of a seven-course bonanza and although Lucas has help from a friend who runs an up-scale catering company, he insists on making one course completely himself and also sourcing all the ingredients. This takes months, although there's never actually a plan – it always comes together at the last minute. Lucas savours the research (and tasting) almost as much as the dishes. It's strange, he wonders, that such small individual plates have made him so big. 'And I am big,' Lucas thinks. 'Becoming the jolly compere is not the look I was after …'.

But Lucas, in his very essence, abhors diets. Just the word makes a shiver run down his spine. Why on earth would anyone eat limp, soggy mung bean patties when there's such a tremendous variety of food available? He just can't bring himself to do it, to count calories or decline a drink when offered. It would be so rude.

In the past, partners have found it hard to be ignored when sincere comments about long-term health have been peppered into conversation. But Lucas is not one 'to be told', well, anything really. His intuition has served him well so far so why should he change?

Food seems to now be entangled with his success and sense of achievement, and he's not sure how or where he'd function without it. Just the thought of 'dieting' makes Lucas feel bereft.

The Gourmet's mind hacks

Because your Gourmet identity is so wrapped up in your ability to entertain and regale, your Shrinkology approach is focused on how to disentangle your deeply entrenched sense of self from the many foodie settings that include indulgent eating and drinking. You will also find a selection of handy quick tips which should help distract you from between meal cravings, as well as great hacks to boost your willpower and see you on the path to success.

DAILY HACKS

How does this serve you?

Gourmets can find it hard to really see why they should change. This poses a bit of a problem as we know that doing it for your own reasons (intrinsic motivation) is a much better predictor of success for any goal than doing it for someone else (extrinsic motivation). Therefore, it's beneficial for Gourmets to work on their inner motivation on a regular, daily basis to help them along their Shrinkology journey.

Whenever you feel that the urge to just do what you've always done (finish off the bottle of wine, order a starter *and* dessert), ask yourself this crucial question:

HOW DOES THIS SERVE ME AND MY HEALTH?

Because of course you can go for dinner and eat rich and heavy, luscious food. You can down a bottle of wine after work with a good friend. You can snaffle all the tasters in your favourite deli. But do these actions serve you and provide you with good health? The answer is probably no.

Passion mind map

You are a passionate person. Although food has become a big part of your passion, it is by no means the only thing you gain delight from. To uncover interests that might have been overshadowed, get a large sheet of paper (or whiteboard if you have access to one) and some coloured pens and sketch out the answers to these questions. There is only one rule: answers must to be non-food related:

- What's the most fulfilling thing you've done?
- What exactly made this so satisfying?
- What gives you lasting satisfaction?
- What have you done recently that you'd like to do more of?
- What are you most proud of?
- What truly makes you feel alive?
- What would you like your legacy to be?

Stand back and look at your scribbles – is there a pattern? You'll notice clusters of life areas – usually in the following categories:

- family
- work, career and money
- living environment
- community
- religion and spirituality
- health and wellbeing

Now take a clean sheet of paper and connect your clusters in a mind map to clearly see where your true passions lie. This may seem obvious, but over time interests can get somewhat lost in the mix of life. Once you reconnect with your non-foodie passions you can invest time and energy on them again – something which, as a Gourmet, you are very good at!

Five mindful senses exercise

To train yourself to become less reactive in food-related situations and gain more control around food, try this mindfulness exercise. It will make the most of your keen Gourmet senses.

- **What can you smell?** Notice the scents around you (ideally not food!) – perfume, a wood burner, or freshly cut grass. Try to identify the individual fragrances.
- **What can you hear?** Focus on road noises, the bustle of a busy office or something more subtle such as the whirr of your computer. Can you hear bird calls, rain drumming on a window or, a cat purring? These are all background noises that we often don't notice on a day-to-day basis. Focus on things you haven't listened to before.
- **What can you feel?** Notice your breathing – sense how it feels to you to inhale and exhale. Do your clothes feel stiff, soft or scratchy on your skin? What's your temperature like – are you warm or a little cold?
- **What can you see?** Take note of colours around you, their brightness and tinge. Try and concentrate on each colour individually before moving to the next.
- **Objects:** scan the environment and find five separate objects to observe. Try to concentrate on each colour individually before moving to the next. Observe five separate objects in this way. It can be interesting to zoom in on the minutiae of an item that you use every day.

By the end of this exercise you will feel calm and relaxed. Remember not to reprimand yourself if your mind wanders – it's simply a case of non-judgementally escorting your attention back to the mindful task.

Crisis control for cravings

Use your remote control

In cognitive behavioural therapy (CBT; page 172) there is a concept called 'frustration tolerance', which is how much you can take before you fall back into old patterns. Because many different situations and triggers have the potential to cause a dieting slip-up, and it's impossible to control every one of these, the trick is to increase your frustration tolerance.

▐▐ When a food or drink craving hits, press the pause button: Now, while your body is in this freeze-frame, imagine yourself giving in to the craving. Be honest with yourself about how the scene normally plays out. Yes, there's the brief gratification, but what else?

▶▶ Next, breathe deeply (see page 189) for a few moments and fast-forward this scene to after you've done this (for instance, about an hour later).

▶▶ Ask yourself now: How does it feel? Are you disappointed to have given in? The guilt, shame and self-recrimination that normally accompany eating behaviour can feel quite strong now. Try not to push these feelings away as they will help you …

◀◀ Now that you have seen the future, press 'rewind' on your remote control and bring yourself back to the present, but this time watch the scene unfold again where you don't give in to the craving. Now you can understand that you're not physically hungry and so you don't need the food or drink – the craving is just a thought.

◀◀ Ask yourself: How does this feel now? Strong, in control and the fabulous person you are? Yes!

▶ Finally, with this increased confidence and empowerment, press play on your remote and make your choice on what you want to do. You have the ability to change the future.

When you're alone

Plan a nostalgia party

You can stick to your weight-loss plan and still throw a brilliant party. It just needs a bit of creativity! Take the emphasis off food and host a nostalgia party. Pick a decade, or even better a specific year, and research the music, movies, games and fads of that particular time. Nostalgia boosts mood and positive feelings about ourselves.[89] Feelings of nostalgia also increase social connectedness, so you'll be able to bond with others over shared memories, rather than wine.

Try these ideas for an 80s themed nostalgia party:

- Make your own *Crystal Maze* with Aztec, Medieval, Industrial and Futuristic Zones. You could stash golden tokens around the house and use the time gained for crystals won in the tasks as the final competition. As the host you will be leading your guests through the Maze's timed games.
- Have a LEGO® competition. LEGO® is not just for kids! There are regular Adult Fans of LEGO® meetings known as AFOL Meetups. Here, people get together and either free build, or work to a theme. LEGO® therapy, originally created to help children with autism improve their social skills,[90] is used incorporate settings to increase confidence and self-assurance (LEGO® SERIOUS PLAY®) and can also help to develop problem-solving skills. But the key is that it's fun!
- Devise a *Ghostbusters* quiz based on all three films, followed by a marathon movie-watching session.
- Throw a *Star Wars* party – the possibilities are endless and not confined to the 80s. But just make sure your friends are fans.

Use scents to stimulate

To replace the stimulation you crave in food and drink, try exploring sensual scents with scented candles, essential oils, herbs, or find somewhere where you can make your own perfume. Blending your own bespoke fragrance enables the Gourmet to later retell the story of your 'signature fragrance/cologne' with as many embellishments as you please.

Quick fix

Boost your feel-good neurochemicals without food

Chocolate isn't the *only* source of the pleasure chemicals dopamine and serotonin – studies show kissing, cuddling and sex can trigger extremely beneficial chemical cascades in the brain too. You can get a dopamine surge (calorie free!) from sex.[91] So, if you are in a loving relationship, why not have more sex instead of chocolate? You get the added bonus of a surge in another neurotransmitter, oxytocin, which is known as the love hormone – this is the chemical which makes us feel warm and fuzzy inside, and connected to our partners.[92] If you're not in a relationship or don't have a willing partner (!) there are other ways to get the benefits of feel-good neurochemicals:

- Kissing is a great way to increase oxytocin and reduce the stress hormone cortisol;
- Reading a steamy novel (try a Mills & Boon series or *50 Shades of Grey*) can boost the brain's pleasure centres;
- Aim to do more hand-holding and hugging;
- Oxytocin is released during masturbation (just so you know …)[93]

Do your homework
(slow-build, longer-term hacks)

Shift your mind-reading ways

The thought of not using food and drink as a conduit for social interaction can feel outrageous and impossible to the Gourmet. You're very likely to start worrying about what people will think of you. In your mind, they'll be saying:

THAT'S SO BORING

YOU'RE NO FUN ANYMORE

YOU NEED TO CHILL

YOU'VE CHANGED

If this sounds like you, you could be engaging in a form of cognitive distortion known as 'mind-reading' in CBT (page 172) and this could be holding you back. We all think we know what other people are thinking, particularly highly sociable Gourmets, but even the most intuitive people are not psychics. And people who say they are psychics are, well, let's just say there isn't a convincing stack of scientific evidence to support this claim. We can't read other people's minds, but we can, and often do, transfer our own thoughts and beliefs onto others. The good news is that if you know you're mind-reading, or rather, guessing, you can stop yourself doing it.

Start by thinking about the criticisms people will inevitably lay at you if you duck out of the heavy eating/drinking social scene and make a list of counter-arguments that support your new, Shrinktastic way of thinking. If none spring to mind, unpick a boozy night out. List the downsides to a heavy night next to the benefits of cutting back a little on the drink (starting with getting rid of some empty calories!)

THE 'FUN' OF A BIG NIGHT OUT

When contemplating a big night out, ask yourself if:
- You'll repeat yourself
- You'll do things you later regret
- You'll don't listen to a word anyone is saying
- You'll get all emotional over nothing
- You'll waste the next day with a hangover
- You'll feel ill and unhappy afterwards
- You'll cancel your exercise session

Now list the advantages of cutting back a little:
- You'll really get to listen to friends and enjoy proper, deep conversation
- You'll wake up the next day feeling refreshed
- You'll have lots of energy
- You won't have a hangover, so you'll have more time for fun
- You'll stick to your exercise plan
- You'll feel clear-headed at work

By challenging your mind-reading thought patterns like this you will increase confidence in your ability to maintain your new, healthier Shrinkology choices.

Experiment, experiment, experiment

As well as challenging your beliefs about how people will react to the new you, it is also useful to collect real-life information with a bit of experimentation. Gourmets are fantastic at experimenting – it's your thing – so approach this method with the same curiosity as you would any new experience. This is all about overcoming health-limiting beliefs that hold you back from being confident about your Shrinkology lifestyle – because what we think might happen in a given situation and what actually happens can be two very different things. Using the worksheet opposite, note down the following:

YOUR PREDICTION: Look into your crystal ball and think about a possible future situation where you are likely to feel a very strong urge to fall back into your old eating and drinking habits.

THE EXPERIMENTAL SITUATION: Think of how you can 'test' (and hopefully disprove) your prediction. Start with something relatively safe where you won't feel too much pressure before moving on to tougher situations.

YOUR RESOURCES: After deciding on the experimental context, gather your resources (work out what you're going to eat, drink and say) before testing the prediction.

THE OUTCOME: After the event, state what happened, including how you felt about it.

YOUR TAKE HOME MESSAGE: This is what you've learned from the experiment – what was the difference between your prediction and the outcome?

Over time and through this 'scientific' method of prediction testing, you will be able to see that even people we think we know inside and out are receptive to your health changes. But perhaps more importantly, you can start to see yourself differently and not be held back by your predictions. Use the table opposite as an example.

PREDICTION	EXPERIMENTAL SITUATION	RESOURCES	OUTCOME	TAKE HOME MESSAGE
If I go out to a favourite restaurant with friends, I think when I get there I'll be handed a glass of wine and when the waiter comes over to take orders he'll assume I'm having my usual. I think he will be stuffy if I don't order the usual and my friends will look on in shock, wondering what's wrong and I'll feel embarrassed and awkward.	It's my close friend's birthday and she's celebrating at a restaurant that we've been going to for years. I love the food there and the owners know me and what I like to eat and drink.	I can speak to my friend beforehand and tell her about Shrinkology.

I know the menu so can choose beforehand.

I can use the booze hacks. | My friend was supportive and asked to borrow Shrinkology! When I got to the restaurant I was quick to order but the waiter actually took no notice at all of the change and the owners greeted me warmly. I still had an excellent time and woke up the next day feeling less tired than usual. | It is possible to still be me with some diet tweaks and a little less booze. It was amazing how positive everyone was about this plan and how many people said they wanted to change their lifestyles as well. |

SHRINKOLOGY SCIENCE: CHANGE YOUR IDENTITY

It is clear that our early life experiences and social context can influence our food choices but could this work the other way round? If you label yourself a Gourmet (or, conversely, a healthy eater) does this make it more likely that you will eat like one? The way in which we identify ourselves has a powerful impact on our behaviour, including the way we eat. The more we identify with a particular role, the more likely we are to carry out actions consistent with that role.

If someone sees themself as an entertainer, they will take every opportunity to try to amuse others, just as a provider will work a tedious job to maintain income. Once defined as a Gourmet, you are very likely to continue through life exploring and sharing your love for food.

But our identities are open to change, even with regard to eating. A study by researchers Amanda Brouwer and Katie Mosack tried to change women's eating habits by influencing their identities.[94] A group of women were asked to create a list of identity statements around their health goals, e.g. if the goal was to eat more fruit, they became the 'fruit eater'. By adding the '-er' suffix to each goal, the participants become 'doers', just as above. In comparison with women given standard nutritional advice or not given any specific information, the 'doers' ate more healthy foods in the month following the initial intervention.

Gourmets can use this approach by noting down health goals and transforming these into self-identities – in other words, if you tell yourself you are a 'small portion eater' you are more likely to become one.

Acting up

Role playing can help you practise challenging situations by providing you with a script as a positive alternative to old habits. Look at your food/mood diary and identify times and situations where the urge to overeat felt overpowering. Remember how this played out and write a script with a different ending. Then, ask a someone to perform this role play with you (or do it alone). It's important to say the words and act out loud as you'll remember it better this way. Even if you don't respond verbatim in similar situations in the future, you'll be better equipped to 'fake it till you make it'. Watch other people to see how they interact with food choices and use these behaviour models in your future role playing.

Gourmet's eat-less tips and tricks

Gourmets are highly resistant to the idea of curtailing excesses in behaviour. You are most likely only reading this book because you have been *told* to lose weight, or you are struggling to find suitable party clothes. Dieting is not a happy place for you and even if previous attempts at weight loss have enjoyed initial success, that sense of deprivation will often lead you back to your foodie passions.

You'll probably skim through the Fundamentals chapter – you know all about *how* to eat properly, and right now you'll be mustering your resistance to fight against any but the most delicious and palatable Shrinkology suggestions. So, if you really want Shrinkology to work, try going back to the Shrinkology Fundamentals and working through them one by one. Just because you really know your cabbages, it doesn't mean the same sensible healthy eating rules don't apply to you.

But here's where your newfound Shrinkology insight is key – now you know the dynamics of your Gourmet traits, and you've seen them in action on the pages of your food/mood diary, you should be ready to take a little bit of well-meant expert advice.

- **Who are you cooking for?** Aim to make a clear distinction between cooking for yourself, with simple, healthy, small, vegetable-based portions, and cooking for others, with a bit more flair and flash. You will not fade away without cold Normandy butter on your crusty French bread every morning, and you can look forward to gourmandising when you cook for friends.

- **Get out your social diary and start pruning.** Fill your days with fun, rewarding activities, but put a self-imposed limit on socialisation that focuses on food. You won't wither away without the positive feedback you get for your curry or crunchy potatoes. If you are going to reach and achieve a healthy weight, you won't be able to do it on more than one food-based entertainment per week.

- **Embrace 'nouvelle cuisine'.** Shrink some of your delicious creations down to bite-sized portions. Exquisite food, particularly when cooked by a Gourmet, can be highly calorific, but life without it is not worth living, so miniaturise instead.

- **Check your food diary.** Are you eating too much of the food you love? You know yourself best. Where can you cut back? Be tough on your self-imposed standards. What highly calorific delight can you more happily live without? Cheese? Chocolate? Butter? Processed meat has had a consistently bad press (the nitrates used as preservative could, if you consume too much, increase your risk of certain cancers). What could you manage without in the long term?

- **Cut out a course.** Would your dinner party be any less enjoyable if you omitted dessert and offered a cheese selection instead (and perhaps tiny petits fours with coffee)? Serve your starter as canapés (thereby blending nibbles with starter and halving the calorific intake). Serve rich desserts in shot glasses or egg cups.

- **Take a look at your values.** Do your children really **need** to be served a gourmet meal every night? Would they love you less if you placed a steaming bowl of pesto pasta in front of them?

- Be snack savvy. Many Gourmets worry about being caught short and hungry, and without access to sustenance between meals. You'll get 'hangry', lack focus, be unable to work or function. This conditioning is partly a product of upbringing (was there always a snack in your school bag, just in case?) and partly the mighty force of the 'Big Food' snacking machine. The truth is, we don't have to snack. Our ancestors rarely snacked. If you eat proper sustaining meals according to Shrinkology rules you will have enough fuel to keep your body and brain ticking along nicely until the next meal.

- Salads and soups are your new friends. Get creative. Flex your gourmet muscle, but ensure one meal each day is a simple salad or a simple homemade soup (with no cream and bulk it up with pulses rather than bread and butter).

- Skip breakfast. It's really not that hard – particularly if you've eaten a big meal the night before. Studies show extending the nightly fast can actually be very good for your health, and that's one very easy way to cut your calorific intake.

- Invest in fab new kitchen gadgets. For instance, a spiralizer could bring you hours of fun as you create lower-carbohydrate (and lower-calorie) courgetti swirls and butternut squash spaghetti, channelling all your gourmet creativity into lower carbohydrate sources of vegetable nutrition. What about a 'vegidrill' which cores fruit and veg in seconds to create fab stuffed peppers, courgette or onions? Or a microwave pressure cooker to rustle up delicious soups and stews super-fast?

GOURMET SOCIAL MEDIA SOS

Social media can be pretty damaging for some Shrinkology types, but as a Gourmet you can, with a bit of judicious selectivity, make some aspects work in your healthy eating favour.

Look out for the latest generation of smartphone apps which allow you to log your daily meals, post photos of your food, and leave comments on other dieters' healthy food posts – it might encourage your tastes away from the most indulgent foodstuffs.[95] Some very clever new apps may even soon use food recognition technology, which determines nutritional information based on photos you upload.

Studies show that for some people, posting your meals on Instagram can be an effective route to weight loss.[96] We think this is a great Gourmet hack. The researchers found that documenting and sharing pictures of your meals using the hashtags #fooddiary or #foodjournal engenders support from other Instagram users and could help you make better food choices. For Gourmets, the Instagram feed works a bit like a social pressure food diary, helping you stay 'honest' and more effectively maintain your healthy habits and lost weight.

The Gourmet's diet digest

For you, food must *never* be thought of as a punishment, so for any diet plan to work, it needs to be able to provide you with joy – ideally more joy than you currently get from the food you love. That's a tough call.

You're certainly unlikely to find long-term success with synthetic meal replacements or low-fat, artificially sweetened diet foods and, for many Gourmets, super-restrictive meal regimes like Weight Watchers or Slimming World aren't sustainable long term. Although you know your 'problem' is the fact that you eat too much rich food, any diet that denies you the chance to cook, feed others and impress, is simply not going to work once you get bored and hit that stubborn weight-loss plateau.

Some Gourmets might find that Atkins-style carb-restricting diets work – for a while. A true Gourmet will be able to push through and enjoy quite a bit of weight-loss success by cutting bread, rice and potatoes out of your diet in return for the hedonistic delight of unlimited fatty steaks, fried breakfasts and thick double cream. But the temptation of triple-cooked fries, fondant potatoes, French bread or a warm croissant with your *chocolat chaud* can soon feel like too much, and extreme low-carb diets are by definition very difficult to modify: you're either doing them or you're not.

All too often the Gourmet will find that coming out of a low-carb regime introduces them to a whole new world of calorific pain, with a stubborn penchant for deliciously fatty foods *plus* the carbs they missed so much on top.

Intermittent fasting might offer a workable long-term solution for you. Some Gourmets can find it much easier to adopt an 'all-or-nothing' mentality whereby they slap themselves with a self-imposed total food ban from after Sunday lunch to, say, Tuesday. Experiment with the length of fast that works best for you. 24–48 hours should be enough compensatory calorie deficit to allow you to eat with impunity – and even enjoy a few drinks – at the weekends. The science shows fasting is also very good for you.[97] Many Gourmets find hungry Mondays (and possibly even Tuesdays, too) are a small price to pay for full food fun at the weekend.

Dr Michael Mosley's 5:2 diet (which allows 800 calories on two 'fast' days and healthy Mediterranean-style eating for the rest of the week) is an option many Gourmets might find worth trying.

Although it can be tough to restrict your calorie intake on two days a week, there are plenty of happy advocates (Dr Mosley included) who use it to get to their target weight, then stay there using 6:1 – sticking to under 800 calories one day a week and eating healthily the rest of the time.

Another fasting diet that might work for you is occasionally eating just one meal a day, as advocated by Dr Xand van Tulleken in his book *How to Eat Well*. He devised a plan which allocates your entire daily calorie allowance to the evening meal. If you keep busy all day and stoke yourself with coffee and tea, it is not the impossible task it might seem. Some Gourmets might find it's a sacrifice worth making for the joy of total unrestrained deliciousness.

If going hungry is too tough, you could try easing yourself in gently with 16:8. This refers to hours rather than days and it is very, very simple. You just have to extend your overnight 'fasting' window and cut your food consumption back to two meals per day. Anecdotally, many people find skipping breakfast is easiest – and research indicates extending your nightly fast can actually be very good for many aspects of your health – so you start the eating part of your day at lunchtime, then enjoy a full sociable dinner. Two meals rather than three.

This will appeal to many Gourmets because they can save their calorie allowance and have a spectacular and elaborate meal with no feelings of deprivation. It's one less meal to worry about and it gets all your calorie restriction out of the way in the morning. It's also a pretty flexible plan. You can try it for five or even six days of the week for active weight loss, or just two days a week to maintain a healthy weight. It can be easily incorporated into holidays and festive periods when everyone tends to eat more than normal.

SHRINKOLOGY SCIENCE: 16:8

Unlike 5:2, which refers to days of the week, 16:8 is all about eating within an 8-hour window. So, if you finish your evening meal at 8pm you eat nothing else until noon the next day. Alternatively, enjoy a slap-up (healthy) breakfast at 8am, and a main meal (lunch or dinner) before 4pm as long as you preserve that 16-hour overnight 'fasting' window.

Studies show continually grazing throughout the day keeps blood sugar levels topped up and insulin constantly storing it away in our fat reserves, so preventing our bodies from using stored fat for fuel. But the theory is, if you give yourself a 16-hour fasting window (during most of which you are asleep) the body will be forced to tap into your fat reserves to keep things ticking over.

Research on fasting seems to show that eating less often could actually boost your metabolic rate and make you even more focused than if you'd eaten a big breakfast.

Gourmet tips to cut back on the booze

Here's the classic Gourmet drinking scenario (to paraphrase W.C. Fields): 'I cook with wine, sometimes I even add it to the food.' Gourmets love food and fine wine quaffed, ideally without restriction, at every available social opportunity.

- Experiment and expand your search for a deliciously exotic non-alcoholic alternative you really like – check out the huge array of choice with an online shop. Stock your kitchen cupboards with exciting options you can share with friends.
- Enjoy a little fine wine, but slow the pace. Put your glass down between sips to slow your consumption.
- Stop and think for a moment – if you struggle with the idea of socialising when sober, could it be that perhaps you're not quite as extrovert as you'd always thought? If you have grown accustomed to using alcohol as a social crutch to drown emotions and calm anxieties it can be tricky to contemplate group activities without it. Cutting back might show you the pleasures to be had in solitude or smaller, sober gatherings.
- Bring out the small 125ml wine glasses that might be languishing at the back of your kitchen cupboard and start routinely using them. Research has shown that when judging the size of a glass we tend to focus on the height of the glass rather than the width and will typically pour 12 per cent less wine into a taller glasses than a wide one.[98] [99] And looking down at a glass makes it seem more full than when holding it, so your top-up will typically be 12 per cent smaller.

The Gourmet's tailored exercise prescription

For the Gourmet to be active it is very important that, as with food, exercise is a joy, not anything that could be regarded as a punishment. This can be tricky if the only exercise you're used to is meandering around the local farmers' market, but it might explain why you find yourself allergic to the gritty tedium of jogging or long-distance cycling which other Shrinkology types might regard as deliciously challenging.

Try channelling your energies into learning a new sporting skill. Investigate tennis or swimming lessons. Learning the ropes and pushing your own limits will keep you entertained. As a Gourmet it's good to feel proud of your body (pride at what it can do as much as pride in how it looks) and proud of your accomplishments outside of the kitchen.

Consider channelling your love of luxury into joining a really smart gym. If the expense seems prohibitive, try adding up how much you spend on wine in a typical month. Cut back, and that gym membership might start to look like good value. It certainly becomes more cost-effective if you absolutely commit to going every other day. And if you're going to do it, do it properly (as only the Gourmet can): use the sauna, the pool, and book beauty treatments too, to make yourself feel pampered and special.

A personal trainer is a very Gourmet thing (it's all part of having and being the best of the best), and you might consider the expense worthwhile initially if you need the incentive to really get started. Halve the cost (and boost the social interaction) by sharing with a friend.

Transfer that Gourmet sense of style to researching and choosing the best possible trainers and sexy new sports kit. If you're serious about increasing your activity levels – and enjoying yourself in the process – it is definitely worth ditching the 'sloth cloth' (that baggy

TRY VINYASA YOGA (YOGA FLOW, DYNAMIC YOGA)

Probably the most widely practised yoga, yoga flow (or dynamic yoga) incorporates a wide range of postures that keep you moving continuously and smoothly. Teachers lead classes that flow from one pose to the next without stopping to talk about the finer points of each pose. Students come away with a good workout as well as a yoga experience.

This kind of yoga might suit a Gourmet best because there's so much room for progression and visible growth (and one day you might be able to impress your friends with a headstand or back bend).

Teachers come up with their own unique sequences, so no two classes will be exactly the same. You'll have the chance to play around with balance postures, inversions, and balances, depending on the level of the class – and everything is suitable for all body types.

It's great if you're easily bored, and it's not too woo-woo and meditative. This practice is also good for those who are looking to feel energised and improve fitness levels.

old T-shirt you wear to polish the car) and investing in some fabulous new fitness gear that makes you feel great while you're being active.

Reward yourself – working towards an end goal with a desired reward can be a great form of motivation for Gourmets. So create your own loyalty system and give yourself a point for every session at the gym. After ten points you can reward yourself with something fantastic (that new bag you have had your eye on, or tickets to an amazing concert).

WEAR MOTIVATIONAL ORANGE

Studies have shown that colours can greatly affect mood, with green being the most calming and yellow being the 'happiest' of colours, but when it comes to gym kit, think orange – it is proven to be the most motivational colour of them all, building energy, motivation and enthusiasm.[100]

Gourmet in a nutshell

Your outgoing and exuberant personality forms a cornerstone of your identity, so the thought of making changes to your socialising and eating behaviours may – at first – feel rather objectionable to you. That's why it's important to boost your other interests and passions to take the focus off any diet plan and to prevent the weight loss process feeling too restrictive or tedious. By taking small steps and making simple behavioural changes, you'll be able to find a little more balance with regards to food and drink. It doesn't mean you're going to have to be boring – instead think of Shrinkology as a wonderful opportunity to tease out aspects of your personality that might have been hidden beneath the cloak of all that food consumption over the years. This could be the start of a great new adventure for you.

If you do one thing …

Before you eat any meal, ask yourself whether the food you are about to put in your mouth is both delicious *and* healthy – these aren't mutually exclusive concepts, especially with your sophisticated palate. The more you can reinforce this message, the better!

Chapter 9
The Magpie

Who is The Magpie?

The Magpie's core concerns are health, happiness and longevity. Many Magpies are addicted to information, particularly information about diets and nutrition. You are always intrigued about the latest dietary trends and you really love to be able to pass advice on. This can at times come across as rather evangelical, but, in fact, you do have a strong set of beliefs that allow you to be idealistic, purposeful, principled and self-controlled.

You could be quite artistic, and even if you don't have a creative job, there's every chance your family think of you as the 'arty one' and you probably make a point of knowing a great deal about art, music, architecture and culture. Certainly your love of research and your fascination with knowledge and information make the Magpie the best travel companion.

Many Magpies are quiet and introspective by nature, but with sophisticated interpersonal skills that allow you to happily dip in and out of many different social situations. Your endless curiosity and quest to gather information make you extremely perceptive and hyper-aware of others, so you're likely to be pretty good at remembering not just someone's name, but also key snippets of their lives they might not even remember revealing to you when you first met. This warms others to you immediately. Having gathered this data you are probably penetratingly accurate in your perceptions of others, and because you genuinely care about the people around you (strangers too!) you might find yourself trying to contribute to other people's sense of wellbeing and happiness.

When it comes to close relationships, the Magpie uses actions rather than words and values the same demonstrative affection in others. Indeed, reassuring words are sometimes not heard to the frustration of partners. You might exasperate your partner or friends by the fact that you demand so much of yourself. In your mind, there are many areas in life that could be improved. To this end the Magpie really needs a little time alone sometimes so you can work through your ever-changing thoughts without interruption.

Your thirst for information makes you a keen trailblazer in many areas (not just food and dieting) – you always know the best books, films and TV shows which is why colleagues and friends come to you for suggestions.

The only problem is that new things come along all the time and you just can't resist the pull of the next big thing ... Your desire for originality and the unconventional is strong, and this can sometimes mean your filter isn't as good as it should be. Once a 'fad' becomes mainstream and everyone's doing it, you are easily bored and you'll be off in search of something shiny and new. In your excitement to take on something new, you might find you sometimes come unstuck.

Classic Magpie eating behaviours

For the Magpie, no matter how entrenched, there's always a shiny jewel of a different dietary regime, extravagant health claims or weight-loss statistics hovering just out of reach. It is a classic Magpie trait to either abandon or adapt your much-loved regime to incorporate your new findings, but in flitting from one dietary regime to another in swift succession you put your body in classic yo-yo diet mode, which sets up psychological and physical changes that can make you a magnet for unwanted weight gain.

You are fascinated by all aspects of health and nutrition. You throw yourself into each eating regime with full enthusiasm and gusto, splashing out on the all-important gadgetry (forceful blender, spiralizer, juicer). Each time you get a new bit of kit or discover a new piece of information you are utterly convinced that this is the way forward and evangelical about it to anyone who will listen.

- Quick to quit. When you start a diet you feel fantastic, lose weight, and your enthusiasm mounts ... but it rarely lasts. You are fascinated by other people's weight-loss success – how they did it, why it worked. On a tough day when the cravings are strong or the numbers on the scales resolutely refuse to fall, your Magpie temptation of another more exciting, potentially more powerful regime can be really great.
- Diet plan mash up. Another Magpie tendency is to use your encyclopaedic knowledge of diets to bend the rules of one regime to incorporate some of another. So you might find yourself kicking off your day with a low-carb breakfast (scrambled eggs with smoked salmon), a superfood smoothie for lunch (packed with fruit), fasting through dinner then bingeing on red wine and nuts in the evening (very Mediterranean). Mixing your dietary metaphors like this can cause nutritional confusion, which means you don't glean any of the supposed benefits of any one regime, and it can leave you vulnerable to super-strong cravings and erratic binge behaviour. It can also lead to a significantly increased daily calorie count, making weight maintenance tricky.
- Too tough on yourself. For the Magpie who holds healthy eating in such high esteem, crazy cravings and off-message feasts can create

a deep sense of disappointment and self-recrimination when adherence flounders. This is not a good state for the psyche and general happiness, and could, in itself, lead to prolonged periods of chaotic and unhealthy eating.

- Too mindful. Whereas most of us pay far too little attention to the food we put in our mouths, Magpies tend to be extremely mindful eaters. This can be a great attribute that can be manipulated to work in your favour. But some Magpies need to watch out for the tendency to analyze every mouthful, self-diagnose minor food intolerances. This can put Magpies at risk of a growing modern condition called 'orthorexia', or the compulsive cutting out of complete food groups (see below).

SHRINKOLOGY SCIENCE: ORTHOREXIA

Experts worry that the popular 'clean eating' craze could be leaving susceptible people increasingly neurotic about food and confused about what to put on their plate. At its extremes, this can lead to an eating disorder called orthorexia – an obsession with defining and maintaining the perfect diet rather than a healthy weight. This can lead to malnutrition and depression as sufferers start cutting entire food groups out of their diet (wheat-based carbs, dairy, sugar, meat) in the belief that these food groups are unhealthy or their bodies are intolerant to them. The worry is that orthorexics could be deprive themselves of essential nutrition and vitamins.

Magpie case study

Mia loves her family very much. She thinks her parents are the best as they have always supported her in everything she's wanted to do. Throughout her life, Mia's family have told her all they want for her is 'to be happy'. And who could ask for more than that? But how can you be happy if no one's told you what this means?

Mia lives in a city and shares a flat with two friends, as they all like to live in a bustling (albeit expensive) area. Mia loves her village-in-the-city as it's swamped with organic cafes, bars and pop-ups. There's always something going on and she often attends seminars, poetry readings and art shows with her friends and colleagues. Mia can see trends before they're even on the horizon and is always ahead of the crowd when it comes to the next big thing. This takes quite a bit of time and effort, though, and it's pretty easy to get rather lost in the detail.

In the same way, Mia scours the internet and travel guides for unique and off the beaten track nooks on trips, she also reads lots of health information. Every day on a bus journey, lunch break or when mooching in front of the TV, Mia will scroll through newspaper and magazine apps which expound the virtues of healthy eating, relaxation, and meditation. She loves self-help books.

And Mia desperately wants to be healthy – because everything you see and hear tells you that health equals happiness, and isn't this what her parents wanted for her, after all? These thoughts about the need to be perfectly happy cascade into even more research and trying new foods and diets to the point where Mia now eats a bizarre combination of different regimes, and weight loss confounds her.

The Magpie's mind hacks

Shrinkology mind hacks for the Magpie will help loosen your preoccupation with health and food trends and release your creative mind to give you a little more freedom to live your life more fully. An important aspect of this is learning to develop self-acceptance and learning to let go of perfectionist thought patterns. It may seem counter-intuitive, but spending too much time focusing on health information, diets, new exercise trends and other aspects of the weight-loss industry (see Chapter 2) can feed body dissatisfaction, low self-esteem and, at its worst, isolation. These hacks will help to break this pattern to give you a properly supported foundation for the long-term health you crave.

DAILY HACKS

Self-appreciation diary

Try this take on a gratitude diary. First buy a lovely diary or notebook – something that you take pleasure from and enjoy looking at. The feel of the diary should also be pleasurable – it should make you feel the same way as a beloved pair of worn out old jeans or tender teddy towelling. Make writing in your diary a happy daily experience – your present to yourself. Set aside time every day to write something you like about yourself, not matter how tiny. This can be something physical, such as the colour of your eyes, or emotional, e.g. what a good friend you are. You can also write memories or anecdotes of times when you felt good. Then, each day before you write something new, read the previous day's entry. Studies show this really can boost mood and happiness, and without deep and fundamental contentment, it's all too easy for the Magpie to search once more for the next bigger, better thing.

Release your preoccupation with health information

Magpies may worry a little too much about their physical health and appearance, which is why you might find yourself trying to grapple with your diet again and again. The problem with this excessive worry is that it can stop you properly enjoying your life. You might find yourself in a self-imposed prison, not constructed from walls and bars but constrained by a stringent regime of information-gathering and body-checking that then loops back into more frenetic searches for reassurance.

You see this loop played out all over social media, and Magpies all too often find themselves getting sucked in. People who are concerned about their health seek out information, but rather than reducing health worries this in fact exacerbates health concerns.[101]

To break free from this cyclical confinement, it's key to first create some awareness of how many times you're checking health and diet information. Then use the hacks in this chapter to help cut down on the number of times you look at this type of info. To help uncover the relationship between health and body shape preoccupation and the frequency of info-checking, use this very simple pencil and paper diary as below:

	SUN	MON	TUE	WED	THU	FRI	SAT
Number of times you paused to read about / view some form of exercise, food, health, nutrition information	42	22	20	12	11	15	18
Preoccupation with health 0–10	10	7	6	4	4	5	5

0 = Not thinking about health at all

10 = Incredibly preoccupied with health, finding it difficult to think about anything else

Now look at your completed table. Is there a pattern emerging? Reducing the number of times you check lifestyle and diet sites will actively dampen your preoccupation with your health. It can be overwhelming to read about a new diet fad every day, as each will do its best to convince it is 'the one' that will bring about perfection and happiness. Therefore, by being aware that this is a negative loop and making the conscious decision that you won't look at your newspaper app health pages first thing in the morning, you can use this time to enjoy life a little more. The fact is our bodies and health are never 100 per cent perfect – as a Magpie you'd like to do everything you can to find perfection, but you'd be far better off doing something fun instead.

Ask yourself this question: what would your 90-year-old self, who's looking back at you right now, say to you about all the time and effort you spend researching food and dieting?

Crisis control for cravings

Fold away the cravings

It is important to try and fill your spare time with mindful activities unrelated to food, exercise and body image, to break your preoccupation with health. Origami is a great way to occupy the flitting Magpie mind, as paper folding develops motor skills, as well as intellectual and spatial abilities. It also makes good use of the Magpie's creative skills. But most importantly, this ancient Japanese art form focuses attention. You will probably want to buy some beautiful origami paper and instruction books but there is no need, just find a piece of A4 copier paper, cut it into a square and make a start with the Samurai Hat overleaf.

Make a Samurai Hat

If you are not using origami paper, make sure the piece you're using is completely square.

1. Fold the square diagonally from corner to corner – if using coloured origami paper, fold with the coloured side on the outside.

2. Now fold each of the two top corners down to the bottom corner.

3. Fold both the left and right flaps up to meet the now top point.

4. Fold these flaps (now in the top half of the structure), along the dotted lines as shown in the figure below.

5. Fold the bottom half up but not all the way, leave about a quarter of the space as per figure.

6. Then fold this strip up.

7. Finally fold back the remaining bottom flap to make the hat!

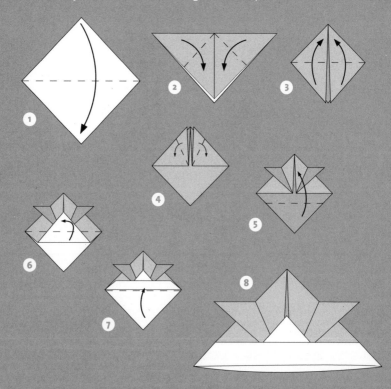

Did you think about eating or food while making the Samurai Hat?

Mindful photography

Mindfulness isn't just a way of thinking – you can also bring a mindful approach to activities. One such pursuit that Magpies might enjoy is photography.

You don't need to buy a specialist camera to do this – you can use the camera on your phone as it's the way you carry out the shot, not the quality of it, that matters. Just one stipulation here: don't use food as the subject!

- Find an object of interest. It can be something ordinary like brickwork or even a common household item like a bookshelf. It's best if the subject isn't active, though, as the purpose here is to look at fine details which can be tricky with a jumping dog!
- Look at it closely. Experiment with different picture angles and take a few shots.
- Observe the minute details. Look at the photo, then choose a detail and try to focus in more on that aspect of the object.

During the photography, you will have thoughts that enter your mind, some of which may be food-related. When one of these thoughts drifts in, acknowledge it, don't fight it. Label whatever comes into your mind as 'a thought' then gently nudge it away. This is an important part of mindfulness. It is not about battling with your thoughts, but rather accepting that your mind will wander and so bringing it back into focus. Just as if an old-fashioned camera was to go a bit blurred, you would notice the distortion, then readjust the lens. Add these photos to your Instagram feed so that it starts to become a library for other, non-food-related interests.

When you're alone

Value your values

As a Magpie you are likely to have a good, strong belief in your own personal values, but you might find yourself overwhelmed because you value so much in life! Problems can arise if you try too hard to live up to these valued beliefs. It can seem impossible to stick to one thing. This is why Magpies tend to flit about and can be prone to feeling overwhelmed.

Self-affirmation theory is a clever device you can use to zoom in on your core values – the biggest issues which really mean the most to you. Practising this exercise will strengthen your sense of self and this could help you to be more selective about the information you take on board.

Studies have shown that by affirming (or validating) your true core values in terms of personal qualities, beliefs or important relationships, you strengthen your sense of self. This can strengthen your self-control in tricky situations and provide you with a buffer against some of life's stresses.

The way in which self affirmations work is via the sympathetic nervous system. Reminding ourselves of our values actively changes the way people experience stress, lowering levels of stress hormones that are usually excreted in difficult situations. As with all the psychological hacks in this book, it helps to exercise this mental muscle so that when stress hits you, you'll be in a more resilient headspace, and won't turn to food as an escape.

EVALUATE YOUR VALUES

1. Rank the list below in order of importance to you (not to your family or anyone else), scoring them honestly from 1 to 11, where 1 is not much and 11 is hugely important.

- artistic skills
- athletics/sport
- business/earning money
- creativity
- independence
- musical ability/appreciation
- politics
- relations with friends or family
- religious values
- sense of humour
- spontaneity/living life in the moment

2. Take your top choice and spend 10 minutes writing about:
a. why this value is important to you
b. a time in your life when this value was particularly important

3. Reaffirm this core value by giving it a score from 1–10 for how much it means to you.

Reinforce the power of this hack by regularly reading step 2 out loud to yourself.

Quick fix

Find your super-power pose!

Body language is hugely influential to everyone and this is a great quick fix for Magpies, who are enticed by health messages in the media. It will instantaneously increase confidence and make you feel more grounded so that you can hold strong to your Shrinkology Fundamentals, ignoring any muddling marketing messages.

- Stand with legs shoulder width apart, feet flat on the ground
- Keep your head up, looking straight forward
- Place your hands on your hips
- Channel your inner Super Hero and imbue strength, force and composure

Studies show that power posing like this for just two minutes is enough to increase levels of testosterone (the dominance hormone), reduce cortisol (the stress hormone) and boost your feelings of power.[102]

Take a ride

Rollercoasters are a great way for Magpies to genuinely 'let go', experience a loss of control, and feel the rush of adrenaline and feel-good endorphins in a safe environment. The excruciatingly slow pull to the highest point of the ride is a great time to put life into perspective – when you get to the top, breathe in deeply and really *feel* the anticipation. This type of safe adrenaline rush helps to overcome fears and increases confidence, especially for those Magpies who are not regular coaster-riders. Also, these will burn calories while 'sitting' (between 40 and 70 calories per ride), tone muscles and even help people pass small kidney stones.[103]

Do your homework
(slow-build, longer-term hacks)

Reality check on perfectionism

While having aims and goals is a positive aspiration, Magpies can be overly perfectionist. Although it is admirable to want to be the best you can, problems can arise if this self-induced pressure leads to frustration and inner criticism. For some, it can result in feelings of anxiety and depression. Perfectionism can also, conversely, cause you to procrastinate or even avoid tasks and activities altogether, for fear of not being able to do them perfectly. This means that life isn't lived to the full; you are at risk of not achieving your full potential through unfounded fear of not getting things right. However, like all limiting beliefs, perfectionism is totally open to change. To start the reality check, have a look at the table below and be honest with yourself – do you fall into the perfectionist side of the table?

	PERFECTIONIST	NON-PERFECTIONIST
BELIEF	I have to be perfect or no one will like me/something will go wrong/I won't be able to get what I need from life.	I am only human so I will invariably make mistakes but this is ok as I can learn from these and move on.
GOALS	I set goals that are unrealistic that are very hard to achieve without significant sacrifice/self-harm.	I set small, achievable goals that are realistic.
FEEDBACK	I give little praise or acknowledgement of meeting small goals. I focus primarily on big picture without positive feedback along the way.	I genuinely celebrate every small achievement. I see how important graduated steps are.
SETBACKS	I see setbacks as utter failure and internalises this by thinking: 'I failed because I am a failure.'	Goal failure means just that – failure to meet goal but not a personal failing.

Now, write down a list of the worst things that could happen to you if you moved to the other side of the table and stopped being a perfectionist. Again, this takes honesty, so note down your true fears, – there is no judgement here.

FEAR	IS THIS REALISTIC?	REALITY CHECK
I'll never meet a partner if I'm not slim.	I know other people who are not slim in happy relationships, so maybe this fear isn't so realistic.	There are millions of people out there who are not slim but who do meet people and fall in love.
If I try to lose weight and then put it back on people will ridicule me.	I know many people who have struggled with their weight and no one has made fun of them for trying.	Many people struggle to maintain a stable weight and so it's more likely that I'll find people with similar struggles than be ridiculed.
If I go to the party everyone will look at me and think how big I am.	Someone may notice my size but it's more likely they will be celebrating with the host.	In general, others are thinking about me much less often than I think about myself.

This reality check can help highlight the overly perfectionist thoughts that might be limiting your enjoyment of life. Use this with the affirmations and daily self-appreciation diary to shift your focus away from unattainable perfection to a deeper sense of self-acceptance.

The Magpie's eat-less tips and tricks

The biggest reason Magpies struggle with their weight is because you rarely stick with any one eating regime for long, and certainly not long enough to become comfortably established into a long-term maintenance phase.

This is partly because many of the most fashionable diets you find so attractive (Paleo, juicing, 'clean eating') can be incredibly difficult and expensive to maintain long term, and partly because the images you find on social media are so impossibly perfect, you can end up feeling as if you're falling short, which leaves you feeling bad about yourself and defeated.

By definition, Magpies get bored easily, and there's always an exciting new diet plan to be researched and tried, so you can find yourself yo-yo dieting your way through all the latest diet trends with no positive lasting results.

They key to finding a long-term healthy, happy weight lies in establishing good, solid Shrinkology foundations which, once in place, will allow you the freedom to play with twinkling elements of new diet plans occasionally, without jeopardising all your best intentions.

- Banish the guilt. Aim to release yourself from your self-imposed stress around food. Life is not one big diet. Food can be savoured and enjoyed. Channel your inner Gourmet and eat the things you deem 'naughty' sometimes too. But don't feel guilty. Enjoy.
- Stop eating food that you don't like. Even if it's portrayed as super-fashionable and super-healthy, life is too short to stuff a mushroom with kimchi, particularly if you don't like kimchi. Experiment with new foods and expand your nutritional horizons, but be honest with yourself about what you like and what you secretly find disgusting.
- Be interested in other things. Aim to channel those Magpie research and fascination tendencies outside of food and body image and into more constructive realms
- Research your research. As a social media aficionado you probably glean much of your information from the web. Magpies are a magnet for crazy health claims and you are likely to stumble upon every outrageous slimming tip and photo-shopped image.

You *know* the web is worryingly unregulated. You *know* this isn't the real world. So make a pact to only read, absorb and share proper *trusted* nutritional research. Remember – anyone can attend a weekend course and call themselves a nutritional therapist. Never follow the advice of anyone without a nutritional degree, and preferably a medical role.

- No more self-diagnosis. Avoid self-diagnosing food intolerances and aim to eat all things in moderation instead. If you know milk and cream make you nauseated then by all means experiment with dairy-free alternatives, but do think twice before jumping on the gluten-free bandwagon, and always consult your doctor.

Should you try gluten-free?

Many people believe they feel better when they cut out gluten. Some medics recognise this as a condition: coeliac lite, or non-coeliac gluten sensitivity (NCGS). The 'free from' sector is the fastest growing in the supermarket, and an astonishing 60 per cent of people are now estimated to buy gluten-free products. Some medics suspect that mild food sensitivities like this can inhibit weight loss, as your immune system treats the food as a foreign invader and then triggers the inflammatory process. This process can inhibit glucose from entering the cells and speed its conversion into fat.

Although cutting out gluten can cure symptoms for some (and you might find you lose weight because you can't just grab a sandwich) you should be aware that eliminating gluten from your diet also removes much of the fibre and some essential vitamins and minerals. A Shrinktastic approach would be to increase the variety of grains you eat to minimise your gluten intake. Don't rely on the 'free from' aisle, as many products are heavily processed with excess sugar and chemicals to make up for the lack of fibre and nutrients.

MAGPIE SOCIAL MEDIA SOS

Magpies tend to relish the multi-layered, ever-sparkling world of social media – you are likely to be a bit of an expert, rarely parted from your phone, with a penchant for photographing your meals and daily rituals. Social media is certainly your main information conduit, but all that time spent online can become distracting, making it hard for you to truly focus, settle or find true satisfaction.

To counter this, it is worth giving a thorough sense-check to your Instagram feed, particularly if the people you are following are portraying some kind of food perfection – either dietary nirvana or the route to perfect slenderness. The 'clean eating' promise of health, wellbeing and effortless slenderness is powerfully seductive for the Magpie but it's not always a good world to be immersed in.

Although a social media overhaul is a good idea whatever your Shrinkology type, for Magpies, creating a blog might be a constructive exercise. Recording your weight-loss journey on a blog could help you identify triggers that make you binge, helping you differentiate between emotional and physical hunger. You can choose to keep it private, or publish it publicly to inspire other Magpies like you. Numerous studies have shown that making a firm commitment to change really can give your mood a boost and can be a real catalyst for change.[104] Once you determine what your triggers are, write about how you'll fix the problem. If you tend to overeat after work, write about what activities you'll do before going home instead. Follow up with notes on how your plan worked.

The Magpie's diet digest

Magpies have little time for fad diets (the cabbage soup or chilli/lemon regimes you might have tried when you were younger) because now you feel you need to be convinced by the research or the celebrity endorsement. You could have dabbled with the idea of becoming vegetarian or vegan, dairy- and/or gluten-free.

You are unlikely to have had much joy long term with complex restrictive plans such as Weight Watchers or plain calorie counting, because they are dull. Similarly, Magpies aren't great fans of meal replacement diets such as SlimFast, as the whole natural food, 'clean eating' movement has been much more bewitching, and you want to keep your body's chemical intake to a minimum.

The key to finding your healthy, happy weight is to channel some of that admirable Magpie research tenacity into reading up about the long-term approaches to your diet of choice. You might be happy whizzing up green juices three times a day, but are you really prepared to sip that piquant kale and rocket broth *every* morning? 'Clean eating' might appear to be a healthy route to weight loss but what about holidays? Entertaining? You need to think if it can last. Before you throw yourself into any new diet plan or decide to follow a new health guru, make a pact to read, absorb and assess the long-term aspects, and consider whether you can commit for life.

The Sirtfood Diet might be good for Magpies. This book, written by two highly qualified nutritionists (Aiden Goggins and Glen Matten) is very science-based and allows you to indulge your love of information (it explores the science of healthy giving plant nutrients called sirtuins – hence the SIRT label), as well as using all the kit (piles of kale and an exhausted juicer) and it is trendy (Pippa Middleton is said to be a fan). There's a short-term, quick weight loss plan which substitutes various meals each day with a home-made green juice of blended kale, rocket and parsley, then a longer-term plan which focuses on eating as many nutritious 'sirtfoods' as possible, plus one green juice a day. If you can stick with it long term your weight should stabilise, which should take the heat out of that Magpie quest for the next best thing.

Many Magpies have concerns about IBS (irritable bowel syndrome). Dr Michael Mosley's Clever Guts Diet focuses on losing weight by boosting your mix of gut bacteria. There's a gut-friendly diet plan which will introduce you to new recipes and foods. This is great if you don't have a lot amount of weight to lose. If you suffer from irritable bowel type symptoms (bloating, flatulence, tummy pain) there's also a special 'repair and reintroduce' plan to help.

It's also worth checking out the Pioppi Principle by cardiologist Dr Aseem Malhotra, which is an offshoot of the Mediterranean Diet. This involves no calorie counting, lots of olive oil, vegetables, fish and nuts.

MAGPIE TIPS TO CUT BACK ON THE BOOZE

The classic Magpie drinking scenario will involve exciting new trends: perhaps a VIP invitation to a newly opened gin bar or a trendy cocktail. Try these targeted tips for cutting back on the booze:

- Shift your friendship get-togethers away from pubs and bars. Nip in first with suggestions of breakfast, where there's less compulsion for alcohol to be involved.
- Factor exercise into your evenings – your new healthy social life that doesn't involve drinking!
- When you turn down a drink, shake your head 'no' – it helps reinforce your decision.[105]
- Add ice to your glass of wine so it lasts longer and is diluted as the ice gradually melts.

The Magpie's tailored exercise prescription

As a Magpie, you might find yourself flitting from one exercise style to another – just as you do diet plans – in your quest for the perfect activity and the 'next big thing'. You may have tried TRX classes, aqua spinning, Piyo (Pilates crossed with yoga), and HIIT, and you'll have let your membership lapse at numerous gyms when the classes lost their thrill.

Although it might seem counter-intuitive, you might benefit from going right back to exercise basics and joining something classic like an aerobics or Zumba class. The key for the Magpie is that a fun, creative and sociable atmosphere is more likely to keep you active on a regular basis than trying to meet that constant quest for something exciting and different.

Aim to move away from any exercise sites on social media, otherwise the temptation to drift back to following trends can be too strong. There are so many hand-standing, back-bending love-lies on Instagram, but yoga gawping is no better than #foodporn as it fuels the devil within.

Search for activities which give you the chance to flex your creative muscle – such as choreographed dance, adult ballet, synchronised swimming or even ballroom dancing. Magpies have such a strong tendency to over-measure and over-research, so this form of exercise can help you learn to be more free.

Conversely, combat training (karate or judo) could help instil a sense of power and achievement that Magpies relish. They key is finding something you are happy to stick at, even if you're not now (or ever likely to be) an expert.

TRY KUNDALINI YOGA

Kundalini yoga probably suits Magpies best. This type of yoga was designed to awaken energy in the spine and classes include meditation, breathing techniques such as alternate nostril breathing, and chanting, as well as yoga postures. It's a slightly unusual style of yoga and you might have to do a bit of research to find a class near you, but it is a great choice for anyone spiritual, as most classes encourage loud breathing and chanting. It is a restorative form of yoga that is healing rather than exhausting. If you can't find a Kundalini class, try Yin Yoga (see Scrambler).

Brief Magpie summary

Magpies love to flit from one shiny new diet plan and exercise style to another, never really getting stuck in but, unlike many other types, Magpies are rather too mindful of what they eat and drink. Your successful Shrinkology mindset should be all about loosening up a little to release your sense of angst and any over-preoccupation with food and health.

If you do one thing …

Stop following Instagrammers who praise overly restrictive food practices. In fact, ease off social media altogether and look away from your phone – there's a whole world out there to be experienced though *doing* rather than *researching*.

Chapter 10
The Rebel

Who is The Rebel?

The Rebel is crazy-sexy-cool. Or at least you were, at some point. You love life and dive eagerly into new experiences – you're a risk-taker, a party-goer. For you if something's worth doing it's worth doing really well. At your most extreme, you might appear fearless, taking risks when others stand quaking. This need for the buzz, the adrenaline, the speed of life means you love to live in the here and now, rarely choosing to put anything off until tomorrow.

The Rebel is lively and fun and enjoys being at the centre of a crowd. You are a great team player, enjoying the camaraderie as much as finding deep satisfaction in working *hard* for the glory of the team. You cherish people and new experiences and you relish excitement and drama in your life. Structure and routine for the Rebel? … Yawwwnnnnn.

As a Rebel, you are not afraid to make a drastic change to your appearance – it's not about trying to grab attention, but more about a love of the excitement that a brand-new look in terms of hair, clothes and accessories might bring.

Rebels prefer to 'go with the flow' and improvise rather than pre-plan. Being decisive isn't an issue but some might think of you as 'hot-headed'. You're not the sort to back down from an argument, and though in certain situations this is great as you don't let others bully you or your mates, this trait can, at times, be perceived as unwittingly confrontational.

For the Rebel, your sense of self-worth is very much embedded with performance. If you run, you run marathons – or triathlons. If you play tennis, you're on the team. It's in your DNA, and Rebels reading this will now be thinking 'yep, and that's a problem why?'. But basing your self-regard on your ability to perform tasks well can cause problems if and when performance is short lived. You might smash your performance goals one day and feel rocketing self-worth, but have an 'off day' the next and wonder why you feel so low.

Also, even when a situation is going well, the Rebel can lean towards self-criticism, which can make you inclined to find *some* fault in your evaluation. Even though you might appear to be carefree to the outside world, you do care deeply about how others perceive you.

The flipside of your fun-loving, devil-may-care attitude can at times be the Rebel's strong all-or-nothing streak. This could make you rather fabulous at short-term diets, but an innate reluctance to be fettered by the hum-drummery of forward thinking could mean that long-term weight maintenance very often gets short shrift.

Classic Rebel eating behaviours

You are the type to throw yourself into a draconian diet or exercise regime with full force, gusto and – often – remarkably speedy success. But (and this is a big *but*) Rebels rarely have a good record for sticking to diets long term, partly because the diets you choose (Paleo, 'clean eating', juicing, low carb) can be complex and very tough to stick with, and partly because, for you, there's no such thing as a small diversion from the plan. You're either on message or you're so far off you're heading in completely the opposite direction.

- All or nothing. The Rebel's black-and-white thinking can lead to a situation where you eat on message, according to strict, self-imposed rules when at home, but go spectacularly off message when invited out, because you manage to convince yourself that here (or wherever) the rules no longer apply. If you fall off the diet wagon, the fall is likely to be spectacular: it's not just one biscuit, but a whole packet, not one beer, but a total bender, not one off-diet meal but a full sit-down Chinese buffet.
- Diet / binge swings. You have a strong tendency to think, 'hey, I'm thin now, I can eat what I want!', meaning you come off the diet, relax too much, then have to go back on a strict and punishing diet which, because your body is so confused, requires you to be even more brutal to lose excess pounds. If this doesn't work, a very typical Rebel fear of failure can be compounded, leading to more extreme diet/binge swings.
- Self-critical nature. You might quit a diet plan before it's had the chance to make long-lasting changes, because your self-critical nature leads you to believe the results just aren't effective or speedy enough.
- Giant-sized portions. If you love sport and regard yourself as a bit of an 'athlete' you could be vulnerable to picking the largest possible portions or going in for second or third helpings because you wrongly believe that 'you can't sustain someone my size on lettuce'.
- Because you deserve it. Some Rebels have a self-destructive tendency towards 'rewards-based' thinking, which leads them to finish off an intense session at the gym with a KFC family bucket (or a super-large latte, a protein bar or hugely calorific smoothie) because you 'deserve it'.

Rebel case study

Raul has had an idea. He will train for a half marathon. By doing this, he thinks, he will lose that extra flab that he keeps seeing in the mirror. He can feel it in the waistband of his jeans. Raul knows he can do it – he's run a 10k and loves his mountain bike, although if he's honest he doesn't remember when he last rode it. But he knows he can lose weight – if he just stops being such a wuss about it.

Raul does really well – he looks online at guides to training for long-distance running and follows them to the letter. This is easy, he thinks. He tells all his friends and colleagues about the training and they spur him on. He buys all the right foods and uses YouTube videos for healthy recipes. And it's working – he feels good about his progress and himself. But then there's a leaving party for a close colleague, and he ends up drinking far too many pints, getting a kebab on the way home and missing his training the day after. That's it, Raul's voice inside his head says, I've ruined it. He thinks there's no point trying any more, it's totally trashed and so calls for a pizza delivery, ordering a family meal, with extras and fizzy drink.

Raul wishes he'd never bothered in the first place now – deep down he knew he'd never be able to do it. All his hard work (in terms of weight loss) is reversed in a matter of days and he feels too ashamed to talk to anyone about the half marathon. This isolation leads to more eating frenzies, and before long Raul is heavier than he was before.

The Rebel's mind hacks

For the Rebel, mind hacks are designed to help break thought patterns that can lead to a massive blow-out. By understanding how your thoughts and feelings can affect your behaviour, and vice versa, you can break these patterns. You should find your fiery temperament will also benefit from immediate craving control hacks, designed to help you snap out of any urgent need to consume.

DAILY HACKS

Going for grey

As the Rebel is an all-or-nothing type of person, your internal monologue (i.e. little nattering voices inside your head) is very black or white. This way of thinking can lead you to feeling overwhelmed, hopeless, anxious and, in some cases, depressed. But studies have shown we have the power to write a new script for our monologues and this really does work – even if you're sceptical.

Practise the simple exercise opposite every day to build your resilience, protect you against feeling too easily defeated and soften some of Rebel's urges for extreme thinking. To take it further, record yourself again or ask your friend/partner to pull you up. Whenever you do use these defeatist or polarised words, add some dosh to a money box that will be given to a charitable cause that you *dislike*. This is a much more powerful incentive than giving to charities we believe in!

By first creating awareness of your use of language you will be able to break Rebel patterns of all-or-nothing behaviour. Instead of saying (or thinking): 'I haven't lost any weight this week, I'm a dieting disaster, I might as well give up,' the exercise opposite will help to re-phrase your thinking to: 'I haven't lost weight this week, but I know I stayed on-plan so I've probably hit a plateau. I will carry on as I know it's helping me to be healthier.'

CONTROL YOUR INNER ZEBRA

First, become your own word detective and sniff out whether and how often you use black-or-white (aka zebra) emotional terms. Use the voice recorder on your phone at different points in the day to capture your natural conversational style. Note down how many times all-or-nothing words tumble out of your mouth. You can also ask a close friend or partner if they think you use the following words frequently:

- ALWAYS
- IMPOSSIBLE
- PERFECT
- NEVER
- DISASTER
- UNACCEPTABLE

Now make a commitment to use softer, kind-to-yourself 'grey' words instead such as:

- SOMETIMES
- OCCASIONALLY
- GOOD ENOUGH
- IT'S OK

Turn 'failure' into feedback

Once you start moving away from zebra thinking, you can also see your so-called failures in a different light. By 'reframing' any perceived failures, no matter how small, through the lens of feedback you'll develop a much kinder and understanding approach to yourself, which will then help to control your characteristic 'what the hell'

mindset and behaviour (i.e. a self-sabotaging binge after setbacks).
Reframing is a great way to turn a negative experience into valuable
and constructive feedback. When your healthy eating efforts don't
appear to be working, don't think of this as a 'diet disaster', instead
ask yourself:

- What have I achieved so far? One diet blip, even a big one, is
  unlikely to undo all the work and time you've invested in the plan
  up until now.
- What have I learned from this slip-up? Were there any specific
  triggers that led to the overeating? Look back at your food/feelings
  diary and see if there's a pattern.
- What can I take from the situation to help move me forwards?
  Can you use some of the tips in this chapter to prevent going off
  course? Do you need more support?

No one – seriously, no one – is perfect. Thank goodness. That would
be so boring. Be honest; the funniest, most engaging stories are invariably based on banana-peel moments. And the best advice always
comes from those who have 'failed' in the past. Speak to people you
know and respect who have achieved goals in their life – you'll find
that their journey wasn't all plain sailing. Biographies of 'successful'
people are also full of the difficulties that they've experienced –
there quite simply wouldn't be a story if it had been an easy ride.

Crisis control for cravings

Rebels can be firecrackers, so it's a great idea to have a handful of
these quick, jolting tips in your back pocket to nudge yourself out of
a craving and get yourself grounded before your thoughts, feelings
and actions can cascade out of control.

You can also ground yourself and in effect halt a binge by:

Shocking your senses:
- Bite into a wedge of lemon. The sharp sourness will send a cascade of messages to your brain, and for l split second you won't be able to think of anything else (taste).
- Ramp the volume on your radio or sound system to 11.
- Pull open the freezer and grab a handful of ice. The extreme cold hurts.

Shocking your mind:
- Pick up a book or magazine and read a paragraph backwards out loud. Reading out loud uses a bigger chunk of cognitive capacity and stops the brain's urge to cheat by skipping over the page to extract meaning from the words.
- Chant song lyrics out loud. Your mind is able to switch off as it focuses in on the next line of the song.

When you're alone

Set realistic expectations

Many Rebels can be a bit pessimistic in outlook and rather self-critical. Sometimes, to the Rebel, it seems like successful people just float effortlessly through life, never facing adversity or, if they do, they respond like super-humans pushing through like some action-movie lead.

But the Rebel, more than any other Shrinkology type, should be aware that summer blockbusters and Instagram feeds don't show the millions of little slip-ups, back-tracking and diversions that make up real life for *everyone*. Social media is without a doubt the worst perpetuator of this, as we tend to only post the best bits of our lives in a polished and preened portrayal of human existence. It's not like that. Not at all.

Life is not a linear journey and things will not always go in the direction we want. This message is tough for the Rebel to accept, but important. You should learn to expect set-backs and slip-ups, and find ways to draw a line in the sand and start the next day anew. Weight loss and maintenance is much more likely to resemble the second graph below, rather than the first. But don't think you need to wait until the next Monday, a shiny new diet plan or any other arbitrary milestone after a stumble – do start again tomorrow.

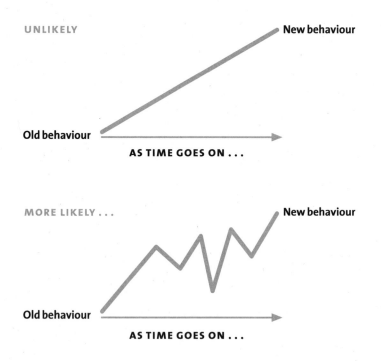

Quick fix

Balance it out

The hot-headed Rebel can use a physical hack to block food cravings. The mind and body are one integrated system, so by doing something that requires physical focus, our thoughts of eating will be set aside. For the Rebel, the 'dammit' feeling is strong but fleeting – after this distraction the overwhelming need to eat junk should have subsided.

> • Start by standing up and facing a wall. Then place your fingers at mid-chest height on the wall and bend your right knee. Next lift your right foot up and balance on your left foot. Remove your fingers from the wall. Try to maintain this stance for 2 minutes while concentrating on a fixed point on wall. Finally, repeat the steps with the opposite legs.
> • If this is too easy, or if you're a yoga-master, try a handstand.

Do your homework
(slow-build, longer-term hacks)

Make a commitment to change

Rebels have no problem with commitment but they do, frequently, have a problem with sticking to it. Go back to the commitments to change you made before starting your food diary: make them your phone background, stick them up around your mirror so they are the last thing you see before you leave the house: whatever you do, make sure they can't slip out of your mind!

Learn your ABCs

No, not the alphabet – instead, how triggers can lead to negative consequences via a set of entrenched beliefs. So:

A = the 'activating event', or trigger that scuppered your diet plan, such as losing an important contract at work.
B = beliefs and attitudes we hold about the activating event, such as, 'I lost the contract and now everyone will know I'm rubbish at my job which is true because I'm no good.'
C = consequences such as anger (emotional) or a fast-food binge (behavioural).

Rebels often blame external factors for their downfalls as they think in an A→C way, completely missing out B. In the above example, losing an important contract would seem to directly lead to a food binge for a Rebel. Once you become aware of your Bs, the activating event might stay the same, but you can change the consequences. To become proficient at our ABC, tweak the B to be more realistic:

A = losing out on a big contract at work.
B = 'This is disappointing but I did my best – some things are outside my control. I'll speak to my line manager about this to see if I can get any feedback on how to manage this type of client in the future.'
C = the emotional consequence is now disappointment and because this is less intense, behaviour is similarly tempered and you will be better able to avoid the diet-busting binge.

It is, of course, easier said than done to simply change long-held beliefs and attitudes, which is why this is a 'do your homework' hack. Like the food and feelings diary on page 62, it is helpful to record events and thoughts around tough events to see our patterns. Try drawing a table like the one opposite:

A – ACTIVATING EVENT	B – BELIEFS	C – CONSEQUENCES
Write down the event or situation that led to 'going off diet plan' or any other behaviour that you might like to change.	Write down your thoughts when the activating event occurred or after it.	Emotions What did you feel then? Behaviours What did you do then?

Another example could be:

A – ACTIVATING EVENT	B – BELIEFS	C – CONSEQUENCES
At a mate's birthday party where everyone is eating.	I think: – 'They'll think I'm boring and no fun don't join in and inhale as many burgers as usual.' – 'I won't be "me" without entertaining everyone.'	Emotions I feel like I'm not good enough and no one will like me if I'm not outrageous. Behaviours I eat 3 burgers and chips and wash them down with beer.

Now, think like a coach again – if your student had written down these beliefs, how would you help them? Challenge your beliefs by coming up with alternatives:

A – ACTIVATING EVENT	B – BELIEFS	C – CONSEQUENCES
At a mate's birthday party where everyone is eating.	I think: – 'Although they might tease me at first my mates will understand that I'm trying to lose weight, appreciate that I've come and not really care if I only have one burger.' – 'There is more to "me" than being the clown.'	Emotions I feel good about myself. Behaviours I have one burger but I'm still the life and soul of the party.

SHRINKOLOGY SCIENCE: CBT

Cognitive behavioural therapy, or CBT, is a therapeutic technique that has strong evidence for its effectiveness. The underlying theory behind CBT is that our thoughts, feelings and behaviour can all interact and influence each other. So, for instance, if someone is a Rebel and they think in an all-or-nothing way, then even the slightest diet diversion will make them feel like their entire weight-loss programme is a complete and utter failure. They not only give up, but throw the towel in spectacularly. The feeling could be failure, self-loathing and/or anger with the accompanying thought of 'well, now that I've screwed this diet up I'm going to have all the foods I've been avoiding', and the resulting behaviour of a massive binge. Then of course the binge triggers more guilt, shame and self-recrimination and thoughts that propel self-sabotage.

CBT uses tools can help people to deal with these 'cognitive distortions' by making them more aware of their underlying feelings and thoughts, as well as challenging these thoughts. This means that behaviours are no longer out of our control as we have the awareness of our thoughts and feelings, the skills to change these thought patterns which then can influence our overt behaviour. CBT can be used to deal with everyday worries or more serious conditions such as depression, anxiety, panic disorder, agoraphobia, social phobia, post-traumatic stress disorder, and childhood depressive and anxiety disorders.[106]

Rebel's eat-less tips and tricks

When it comes to eating, the Rebel swings hot and cold. You're either being spectacularly efficient and achieving success, or you are way off message and eating unhealthily, possibly even vowing never to diet again.

Your food/mood diary might be a revelation to you, and a glance through the Shrinkology Fundamentals should give you food for thought. These targeted nuggets of advice might help to smooth some of the excessive peaks and troughs of your dietary rollercoaster.

- Create your own 'respite plan'. The Rebel will normally kick back against future planning. For you, it's all about the here and now. But you can take steps to protect your future by building yourself a happy middle ground for the times when weight loss seems like an insurmountable climb. What you need is a framework for a kind of dietary halfway house which won't trigger weight loss, but can be your safe and healthy eating place when times are tough and a diet plan is the last thing on your mind. It is here to stop you blowing your best intentions, bingeing on the foods you've denied yourself, and catapulting yourself back to the start with self-recrimination and despair.

- Try intuitive eating. Food rules can lead to binges when they're broken. Instead of trying to keep up with the latest 'carbs are out' or 'kale is in' diet rules, try this technique whereby you eat whatever you want, but only when you're hungry, and stop eating as soon as you feel full. By really focusing on your food choices and being hyper-aware of any cravings, urges and hunger pangs you can start to re-condition your sensors and allow your brain's natural energy-balance system to slip back in control. It may take time but 'intuitive eating' works with your brain, not against it, teaching your body to eat in a way that's relaxed and satisfying so your weight can settle at a comfortable level and stay there. Long term.

- **Create your own insurance policy.** This is your 'go-to' strategy for the times when everything goes wrong. Take a few quiet moments to think about exactly why you want to be achieve a happy, healthy weight. What are your true drivers? Jot them down on a coloured card, or attach a picture of someone you hold dear, to whom your quest for long life and vitality can be dedicated. This is your 'brake in times of emergency' prompt. So when you find yourself starting to teeter on the edge of a deliciously tempting dessert menu, STOP. Pull out your emergency card for a stark reminder of why it's worth saying no this time.
- **Turn up the volume on 'real food'.** Rebels can be suckers for a 'low-fat' or 'low-sugar' label and you might find it tempting to fill your shopping trolley with foods endorsed by 'winners' (celebrities) or which purport to promote strength and vitality. But these can be surprisingly unhealthy and calorific, particularly if you are inadvertently consuming far more calories than you expend in supposedly healthy protein shakes, energy balls and sports drinks.
- **Stop reading and get going.** The Rebel learns best through 'hands-on' instruction, through 'doing' and interacting with others rather than by reading a book (unlike other Shrinkology types), so investigate healthy cookery programmes and inspiring YouTubers (such as Joe Wicks). You might find a healthy eating cookery course at a local adult education centre.
- **Think marathon, not sprint.** Maintenance is key to preventing the extreme yo-yoing patterns that Rebels can so easily fall into. Aim to shift your mindset from a sprint mentality to a marathon. You know you like challenges, so after your initial weight loss, set future goals so weight doesn't creep back on. Start with monthly goals and progress to a yearly weight check. When you arrive at each goal refresh your Shrinkology Fundamentals to ensure you're still sticking to these basic principles.

Rebels thrive on feedback so you might find it useful to put your weight-loss goals on social media, and keep track of the 'likes' (in a typically Rebel competitive way). Studies have found it can make you more likely to stick to your intentions too.[107] Researchers believe Twitter can be an effective weight-loss tool for some people, because it provides increased access to information along with accountability and potential social support. Another study assigned one group of adults to listen to two nutrition and fitness podcasts each, and another group to listen to podcasts in addition to reporting workouts and connecting with other study participants on Twitter. They found that every 10 tweets in the second group corresponded to a 0.5 per cent greater weight loss.[108]

The Rebel's diet digest

As a natural risk taker, you prefer the sort of diet and exercise plan that gives you adrenaline and buzz, but the more complex the diet plan the more likely it is to set you up to fail with the attitude that if something is not completely right, there's no point doing it at all.

The Rebel will have tried – and *loved* – Atkins and Paleo and you are likely to have thrown yourself in with gusto, and to have had fantastic results . . . for a while. You love the extreme nature and the competitive tang and 'this is *not* a diet' glory of being able to sit down to a huge T-bone steak and buttery cabbage, or pouring thick cream into your coffee. But for the Rebel, these diet plans are hard to sustain. Your extreme nature feeds the Rebel's most extreme tendencies. Psychology matches biology. On a bad day the Rebel might steal chips off their partner's plate and think 'noooo! My diet is lost' and the infuriating truth is, if your body is happily using fat for fuel, that sly extra chip could tip you back into fat-storing mode. If you love Paleo and Atkins, then the key to success for the Rebel should be – from now on – to scrutinise the long-term plan first. Can you live without bread and serve up steaks for breakfast long term? Dial the whole process down, take yourself out of the short-fix crisis mode, and work out a way to incorporate the important principles into your life long term. Aim to keep food to a steady plan. Food and diet should shift to the back burner. Turn down the volume to stop that part of life being 'a failure'.

Any repetitive, rigidly structured plan is doomed to fail because, for the Rebel, if something's not fun, it's not worth sticking to. Some Rebels might see success with organised slimming groups such as Weight Watchers or Slimming World, which might appeal to your sociable nature and give the opportunity for regular feedback in the form of the weekly public weigh-in. But other Rebels might find the dietary regime insufferably restrictive. Intermittent fasting, such as 5:2, is also unlikely to work long term because you will – for sure – balk at the rigid structure and the sheer grind of those two fasting days. Similarly, you'll have had little joy with cabbage soup or lemon/cayenne pepper or bone broth because of your low boredom tolerance. If one thing is for sure, you can't give a Rebel boring food and expect them to be happy.

The Sirtfood diet might appeal to the Rebel because it's glamourous and full-on (Pippa Middleton apparently credits it for her sinewy arms and abs) and there's a manageable longer-term option: you can go hard with the juicing phase, then drop back – not abandoning the whole thing and catastrophising, but eating instead from a list of 40 nutrient-packed foods – and return to the weightloss juicing phase a little later (see page 156 for more details).

One meal a day (the Dr Xand van Tulleken plan – see Gourmet for more details) could work well for you because it requires you to command that steely Rebel willpower during the day, then concentrate all your eating efforts into a nutritious and sociable meal in the evening where you need little constraint. This makes the most of the Rebel's 'all-or-nothing' mentality.

Extreme meal replacement diets (such as Lighter Life or SlimFast) might give you a quick success but that's because they are extreme and you'll be relishing the feedback from seeing those numbers tumbling on the scales. But for the Rebel, this kind of food restriction is rarely sustainable long term. If you have a lot of weight you want to lose, and this has been recommended as an option, just make sure you have your exit route clearly marked when you start. You might think you'll stick with it until you reach your target weight and worry about future eating strategies then, but it's important to factor in the Rebel glitches – those moments when you come unstuck, the plateaus, the impossible-to-resist 'escape' opportunities – and have a secure, manageable long-term plan in place.

Read ahead to the long-term maintenance plan of any diet so you know where this is going. If that seems unfeasible (and for the Rebel it might), borrow a long-term strategy from another diet plan and aim to go with that.

Any diet plan you choose needs to be very goal-oriented and results-driven so you can measure your success (on an on-going basis). Weighing yourself regularly is crucial for the Rebel, keeping in mind that progress isn't always linear and tips to deal with times when the scales don't tip in the preferred direction. See page 172.

The key, for the Rebel, is sticking at something – anything truly enjoyable and sustainable – long term. And your diet plan must be *fun* – Rebels love to bring others along on their fun rides and you are typically a lot of fun to be with. If the diet and exercise aren't fun, you'll never stick to them.

Rebel tips to cut back on the booze

Rebels can be highly vulnerable to drinking to excess, and these include beer binges or the all-or-nothing, drink-to-oblivion Big Night Out. For the Rebel, the art of cutting back, or cutting down on alcohol, has to be approached with a delicate touch, so try these tricks:

- Have a small list of delicious non-alcoholic drinks you like and be absolutely ready when someone asks: 'What do you want to drink?' Rehearse your no-booze order by repeatedly saying it aloud. With conviction. It's a good idea to have a second and third option lined up to prevent you from defaulting. By rehearsing healthy routines over and over you harness the power of visualisation to re-programme your brain and establish healthy habits.
- Do an online shop and stock up your fridge with no-alcohol beer and wine. There is a wider choice available than you probably realise and they look the same and even taste pretty similar when nicely chilled and poured into the appropriate glass.
- Don't wait for Dry January or StopTober, make drinking less – or not at all – a competition. Pick a worthy charity, pledge your drinking money for a month and get the office or friendship group involved.
- As a Rebel you're more likely to be a 'starter' than a 'stopper', which means once you start drinking you find it very hard to stop. So aim to start on soft drinks with the option of switching to something a little stronger later in the evening.
- Get your order in first. If you're out with a group, it's much harder to be the only one ordering water when everyone else is on the wine, but if you get in first with your soft drink order there's every chance others will be relieved and follow suit.

The Rebel's tailored exercise prescription

The Rebel is very often a great team player, and exercising in a group is a fantastic way to capitalise on your strengths. Why not get together with the football gang or the tennis club to reach competitive exercise goals or sponsored challenges? You'll be far happier channelling your extreme tendencies into sport than a diet because 'failure' is less likely to lead to self-destruct in the form of chaotic eating. However, Rebels would be well advised to avoid letting their chosen mode of exercise define them. Take a tough spinning class, intense boot camp circuit training, join a cycling club, but watch out for the Rebel inclination to want to be the best, and the tendency to cave if you're not.

Group sports are a must as the Rebel finds group support just as important as working *hard* for the glory of the team. You are the type to really benefit from the self-worth you might get from working with others (to take the focus off yourself), so ask about a local football team or cycling group.

The Rebel is adventurous and seemingly fearless. Indulge that trait and have a go at every 'extreme' experience you can find (bungee jumping, Zorbing, jet ski, etc.).

If you can pick a sport with a competitive spin (like a results-oriented spinning class), then you'll certainly find that more exciting and therefore stick to it as you battle to stay at the top of the leaderboard. Book a course of classes and pre-pay so you have a financial incentive to keep going through the ups and downs in your sporting performance.

Fix a longer-term goal, a slower burn, and one that is less likely to set you up to potentially fail, such as a tennis ladder (as you improve you work your way up) which you can combine with lessons (to hone those admirable sporting skills).

Consider putting yourself up to coach a team so you can channel your sense of achievement into others. This could be key to achieving the self-esteem you need to maintain a healthy weight and body image. Directing your energies and your passions to help others will act as a perfect foil, taking away the urge for self-focus.

You can be intense and you tend to be externally motivated (driven by a sense of competition) so you are likely to respond well to specific training plans to reach personal goals. Try High Intensity Interval Training (HIIT, see page 209), spinning, cardio conditioning or triathlon. Your need for results can leave you impatient and frustrated at times, so a very specific, time-sensitive and action-oriented approach to exercise works best.

TRY ASHTANGA YOGA

Rebels will either love or hate the idea of yoga, but if you're going to try one type, let it be Ashtanga. This style is much loved by competitive, ambitious type A personalities who like a challenge and a set routine. As you progress you feel great pride in being able to achieve postures and balances you never knew you could do. Ashtanga is a more vigorous style of yoga. It offers a series of poses, each held for five breaths with sequences punctuated by a half sun salutation to keep up the pace and heart rate. You are expected to memorise and follow a set sequence of postures that get progressively more complex as you move through six different series. It is great for building upper body strength and general fitness – like circuit training on the yoga mat.

Brief Rebel summary

Rebels can be amazingly disciplined but when something goes a little wrong, you are also quite spectacular at throwing in the towel. The key to true Rebel Shrinktasticness is to nudge yourself away from zebra thinking, and understand that you can still achieve health and fitness on a less extreme regime. By being more realistic about your dietary goals, you're actually more likely to be able to stay on track. You're only human after all …

If you do just one thing …

When you feel things start to slip, STOP, let it go and move on. Long-term health change is not a smooth, linear progression, so expect some blips and use your personalised tips and hacks to get back on plan.

Chapter 11
The Scrambler

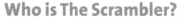

Who is The Scrambler?

The Scrambler is busy, busy, busy. You're always on the go, juggling tasks, spinning plates and squeezing more into one day than many people manage in a week. You're the classic 'I don't know how they do it!' person. Of all the Shrinkology types, being a Scrambler is less about emotion and personality and more about circumstance. When you have a young family, for instance, and suddenly babies and children have to be shoe-horned into your already busy life – that's when any Shrinkology type can start to scramble. Scrambling can just as easily describe the ambitious worker trying to fill every snatched moment with tiny snippets of the rest of their life between long, long hours at the desk and 24/7 email connectivity.

Despite everything going on in your world, Scramblers rarely feel put-upon. In fact, most of the time you are happy to juggle. It might be madness, but you secretly love teetering on the (right) edge of chaos and the buzz of constantly bubbling stress. Without it you suspect you'd be bored and you get restless if every minute of your day isn't high paced and high pressure.

You're a great team player because you have the innate skill of being able to keep everyone's strengths and weaknesses in mind, ducking and diving and going with the flow when and where needed. You are by necessity highly organised and will always know where everyone needs to be and when – although sometimes it may feel like you get there by the skin of your teeth.

The Scrambler is most definitely a 'doer'. If you can avoid reading a whole book when you can flick through it, you will, or watch a YouTube video instead. You might come across as being extremely confident, capable and in control, but some Scramblers harbour a secret fear that they might be a bit of an impostor and not actually good at anything. You can also be bothered by the constant niggling fear that you might have missed something (though you rarely do).

Underneath your super-efficient surface, your legs will be paddling furiously to keep it all going. The Scrambler tends to think about a million things at once, and because you are so adept at multi-tasking you have a mental rollercoaster continually running in your head. This can make for a hairy ride (when you realise you really do have to be in two places at once, say), which isn't always fun. The scattergun approach means your thoughts can wander, plates can come crashing down, and the never-ending effort of holding everything together can leave you feeling utterly exhausted at the end of the day.

Even though Scramblers are intelligent, competent, caring, protective of those they love and utterly dependable, you're not great at receiving and absorbing praise. Instead, many Scramblers might find themselves plagued by the feeling that you can and should do more; do better; do it all, and you probably rarely give yourself credit for your many achievements.

With so much going on, the Scrambler can find it extremely difficult to eat healthily and exercise regularly, and your weight and health can suffer. But your life has umpteen moments of laughter and joy and is packed with truly special memories – if only you could just press pause for a moment to properly enjoy it.

Classic Scrambler eating behaviours

Scramblers tend to pick at food – you're the sort to prop yourself up with coffee and adrenaline, skip meals and mindlessly grab snacks to keep you going throughout the day. It can be easy to convince yourself you've eaten nothing, but those snack calories can soon to add up.

- Snack happy. Your diet of sugary snacks and grabbed convenience food is nutritionally poor and very likely to set up cravings for more high-fat, high-sugar, quick-fix sustenance. When you've rarely time to shop for, prepare and sit down to eat a balanced and nutritious vegetable-based meal, processed food becomes an unhealthy lifeline.
- Wind-down wine. Many Scramblers depend on a 'medicinal' glass of wine to help at the end of a long day. It is your 'reward' for a job well done. But every glass is packed with empty calories and the alcohol can weaken your resolve, making you less likely to resist crisps or pizza (not to mention the bowl of sugary cereal that you 'need' in the morning to get you through the grottiness of a restless, booze-infused night's sleep).
- Back-loaded days: If you use adrenaline and caffeine as props throughout the day you are likely to find yourself extremely hungry by the evening and prone to 'back-loading' your day with indiscriminate eating of an abundance of unhealthy foods.
- Lacking nutrients. You rarely keep track of your nutritional intake so you are likely to be nutritionally depleted with a weakened immune system and vulnerability to every cold and bug going around.
- Relying on energy props. You're likely to use sugar and caffeine to get you through the mid-afternoon energy slump – but these only artificially hike your energy levels, often dropping you in an exhausted (and hungry) slump by evening.

- Fragmented sleep and/or working late into the night. This could put you at the same risk of health problems and weight gain known to frequently affect shift workers.[109]
- Time poor. Your chaotic, stressful life makes sticking to weight-loss diets super-tricky (do you have time to whip up a green juice or separate your egg whites? I don't think so!), and this puts you at the perils of yo-yo dieting (see Chapter 1).
- Eating on the go. When you do eat, you eat **fast** and usually while doing something else. This means your brain struggles to register the fact that you are eating, and your body never gets the stress respite it needs to effectively digest your food.
- Restricted healthy options. If you're a working Scrambler, circumstance might mean you are tethered to the nutritional peccadilloes of the office canteen, the meeting room sandwiches and the regimented boardroom coffee and biscuits.
- Too much temptation. For parenting Scramblers, hunger, tiredness and willpower hanging by a thread can mean the bountifully stocked 'snack drawer' and fridge groaning with high-calorie, child-friendly treats are impossible to resist.

Scrambler case study

Claire is frazzled. But isn't everyone? Claire doesn't know anyone who isn't juggling work, family, parents, kids' activities and oh, wait a minute, trying to maintain some sort of semblance of a relationship. But somehow everyone else seems to keep it all together a little bit better while rushing, fitting everything in and over-scheduling. Not that she's complaining – Claire loves to be the cornerstone of her family, the go-to person at work when a leaving party needs to be organised and she would never (ever) miss a parent–teacher event. All the aspects of her busy life make Claire feel truly alive and she wouldn't want to give anything up – it would just be nice to have a few more hours in the day, that's all.

It's also pretty damn frustrating that she feels like she never quite does anything properly – as a parent, in her career, as a friend, as a partner. Sometimes she feels like a bit of an impostor and wonders what will happen when everyone finds out she's just been winging it all along. Claire has a low-level but genuine fear that she'll drop the spinning plates, and everyone will know the real Claire, not this fake Claire that manages to do everything somehow. And then what will happen …?

Claire does know that something's got to give. Somehow, somewhere, the importance of self-care has become lost in the whirlwind headspin of life. Claire doesn't remember the last time she thought about her own needs – there are always more pressing issues and 'it's ok,' she thinks, 'I'll get back on track with diet/exercise/myself after I sort out this mini crisis.' Of course, this time, the moment when everything freezes in mid-air, is a fantasy – the world doesn't stop spinning, especially as Claire is the one turning the wheels.

The Scrambler's mind hacks

For the Scrambler, the key to really making Shrinkology work is to use clever mind hacks to help convert you from a 'human doing' back into a 'human being'. It can be all too easy to equate who we are with what we do – what we do for work, what we do for other people, what we do online … But, in the quest to be truly healthy, it is worth taking a moment right now to stop and think about how much of your day you spend actually 'being'. This doesn't mean sitting perfectly still in a meditative pose, it's about pausing, just briefly, to clear your head and just be, rather than continually thinking about all the other things you should and could be doing.

Here you'll find Shrinkology mind hacks designed to help you be a little more mindful throughout your day, and also a targeted selection of very clever and research-backed techniques to help destress your mind and body. Stress can lead to physiological changes that drive us towards unhealthy eating patterns (Chapter 2); by using Shrinkology hacks that fit into your life you'll be able to reduce stress and prioritise yourself just a little more mindfully. Approach them all with an open mind, then cherry pick the ones you like best to work into your own personalised weight-maintenance plan.

DAILY HACKS

Scramblers live life at a high speed so the thought of adding in 'yet one more thing' can just add additional stress, but it is possible to sprinkle short bursts of mindfulness into your day without specifically scheduling sessions into your packed diary. The key is cleverly using everyday activities or thoughts as an anchor for simple mindfulness exercises.

MINDFUL ANCHORS

- First of all, choose a simple action you do multiple times day (boiling the kettle, putting on your shoes, getting into the car) to be your 'anchor'.
- Now, whenever you find yourself about to do this 'anchor' activity, stop yourself before your mind starts jogging through your to-do list. Instead, take out your mental torch and shine a metaphorical light on this moment in time: where are you, what are you about to do?
- Now ask yourself (internally) how you feel right at this moment. What physical sensations can you feel? The hard back of a chair? The feeling of your socks and shoes on your feet. What can you smell? Hear? For a few seconds, pay close attention to any sensations you might normally overlook.
- Take a very brief moment to stop here with these insights and breathe deeply.
- If a thought pops into your mind ('I must remember to stop off at the bank', or 'do we have carrots for supper?'), acknowledge it, label it as a thought, and softly nudge it aside.

Using your 'anchor' to trigger these brief moments of mental respite means you will – without even really noticing – be peppering your day with mini mindfulness episodes. Very quickly this will help to break that constant 'wired' feeling by slowing down your internal pace. With practice, this technique will help sharpen your focus so you can concentrate more fully on each task rather than tripping over yourself to get on to the next one without giving the first the attention it really required.

Deep breathing

When we are young, we naturally breathe from the belly, but when we are busy or stressed we tend to breathe from the chest, and the habit can become ingrained through poor posture, ill-fitting clothes and even the desire to hold our tummies in. Quick chest breathing is also a characteristic of the stress response, and at its worst can contribute to hyperventilation and panic attacks. Deep breathing, on the other hand, dampens feelings of anxiety and stress.

Re-learning and focusing on breathing like we did as children, by properly engaging the diaphragm (a dome-shaped muscle lying beneath the lungs) is a very simple way to destress quickly. Breathing through the diaphragm reduces the stress response as it triggers the parasympathetic nervous system, which helps us to regain equilibrium.

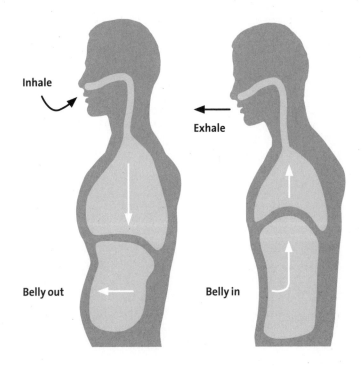

Inhale

Exhale

Belly out

Belly in

ARE YOU REALLY RELAXED?

This exercise can be done any time and any place to bring an instant feeling of calm but do factor it into your day at least once, for example every morning just before you get out of bed or in the evening after you brush your teeth. You can also practise this exercise at night to help reduce any tension prior to sleep. Here's how:

- Start by asking yourself: 'On a scale of 1–10 how relaxed am I?'
- Now locate your diaphragm. Put your right hand on your tummy and place your little finger just above your belly button. Your diaphragm is directly under your palm.
- Next put your left hand palm-down on your chest.
- Inhale at a slow and steady pace through your nose for a count of three, noticing the hand on your belly rise up as you draw in air.
- Exhale at the same pace for another count of three and feel your right hand dip down with your belly towards your spine while saying the word 'calm' in your mind.
- During both the inhale and exhale your left hand on your chest should be still – if it's moving up and down take a moment and then try again, concentrating on drawing the breath down into your belly.
- Repeat 5–10 times and check in with yourself on how you're feeling by asking, again on a scale of 1–10, how relaxed you are. Using this tiny evaluation will help motivate even a busy Scrambler to take a few moments to breathe.

Crisis control for cravings

Free cravings with tapping

There's a great self-help hack called 'Emotional Freedom Technique' (EFT) which requires you to tap lightly on various points of your face and arms. It might seem bizarre and kooky, but EFT has been researched scientifically and it is particularly useful for Scramblers because it is a quick method that can be used on the go.

While many people use EFT to relieve stress and pain, it has been shown in research studies to curb cravings.[110] The theory behind this is that tapping acupressure points around the body helps to 'unblock' any obstructions in our energy meridians. Certainly the affirmations (positive self-talk) can help boost our ability to cope with strong desires for certain foods. Try it and see what you think:

1. When a craving strikes, rate its intensity on a scale of 1–10 (1 = not at all strong, 10 = as strong as it could possibly be).

2. Choose one of these affirmations (or invent your own):
   - I am able to cope with these cravings and nudge them from my consciousness.
   - Even though I have cravings, I accept myself deeply and fully for who I am.
   - Although I doubt that tapping works, I completely and truly love and accept myself.

3. Now find the 'karate chop' point on the outer edge of one hand (see page 192). Using the index and middle fingers of your other hand as your tapping tool, tap this area five times while breathing deeply in and out (once) and silently repeating your affirmation.

4. Repeat the process on each of the points below (it's easier than it sounds after the first try – if you find you're concentrating too much on your breathing leave this out for now):

- inner edge of the eyebrow
- outer side of the eye
- under the eye on the bone of the eye socket
- under the nose where it dips
- on the dip of your chin
- on your collarbone, slightly in from the sternum
- under the arm, about 10cm down from the armpit

5. End the round of EFT by:

- tapping the inside of both wrists together
- tapping the top of your head with a the flat of your palm

6. Finally, score from 1–10 the strength of the craving.

EFT TAPPING POINTS

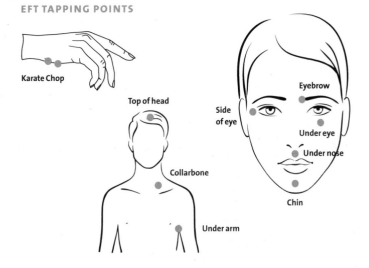

With a bit of practice, this technique is very quick. If your craving score didn't reduce, you may want to do more than one tapping round or change the affirmation to something even more specific to you.

Smile

Researchers have found that even manufactured smiling decreases stress[111] but real smiles that use the muscles around the eyes and mouth work best. So when a craving strikes, flash a fake 'Joker' smile, or, better still, think about something funny and put a proper smile on your face.

TRY FLEXIDESKING

If you just haven't got time to get to yoga, try these exercises you can do at your desk or the kitchen table:

- Spinal twist: sit straight, looking ahead with your chin parallel to the floor. Breathe in deeply through your diaphragm. Then, as you exhale, twist from your abdomen to the right. If you have an arm rest on your chair grasp this, if not, hold your arms out to the side. Maintain this pose for a count of five before returning to the centre. Pause here for a count of two before twisting to the left.
- Reach for the sky: straighten your spine. Inhale deeply and lift your arms to the sky, with your palms facing inwards, fingers stretched. On the exhale, gently draw your chin up so you look to the ceiling (bending from the upper back rather than tipping over). Count to five, then slowly bring your arms back down to your sides. Repeat three times.
- Anti-hunch: first, move your chair out of the way and then stand a few paces back from your desk. Breathe in and slowly bend so that your fingertips are touching the edge of the desk. Let your head fall gradually in between your shoulders. You should feel a good stretch in between your shoulders.

When you're alone

Take a mindful shower – literally

Another way to fit a bit of mindfulness in is in the shower or bath. The key here is to fully attend to the small, mundane, details of a shower. You could use any day-to-day task – washing up, folding clothes, making a cup of tea, etc. If you've ever taken a shower and not remembered if you've washed your face yet, this one is for you.

- **FOCUS.** When you step into the shower, focus your attention on the temperature of the water.
- **ACKNOWLEDGE.** If, at any point, your thoughts start to slide into 'to-dos' for the day, note them, tag each thought as 'a thought' and gently push it away (with time and practice, you'll have fewer gliding thoughts but it's completely fine if you have many – there's no judgement here).
- **NOTICE.** Now, when you start using the soap or shower gel observe how it foams in the water. How do the bubbles feel on your skin? Give yourself a brief moment to observe this sensation.
- **FEEL.** Observe the spray of the shower now. Let the water drip on your face, especially as this can mimic tears (see page 222).
- **TURN INWARDS.** Take your mind to how your muscles feel. Observe how the tension slips out of them and merges with the water as it drains away.
- **BREATHE.** Before you get out of the shower, check in with your breathing and see that it is now regular and deep.

A shower is (usually!) the one place we can be alone and take a few minutes to be mindful. You'll be surprised how every day you can notice new sensations in this completely ordinary activity. Depending on when you wash, this will either set you up for the day or relax you for a good night's sleep.

Try a little 'worry work'

Worrying can consume a lot of mental energy and lead Scramblers to graze on food and drink throughout the day in an effort to dampen negative mental chatter. But by allocating and ring-fencing a time slot to constructively tackle worries each day, you'll be able to concentrate on individual daily jobs which will not only help to manage stress levels, but also add an increased control to your life.

This daily hack separates out any worries and allows you to deal with them separately so you can better focus your attention on your everyday jobs. All you have to do is set aside five minutes at the end of each day to deal with any niggles or concerns. You'll need to dedicate a special notebook or a file on your laptop for worries, then make a neat list of all your concerns, be they practical, emotional or if there's just a general nagging feeling of unease.

At your designated 'worry' time each day, take out your notes and see if those worries are still a concern, then, if they are, address them in the following way:

1. Jot down options to help you deal with any practical concerns, such as organising the children's half-term childcare. You don't need to have all the answers to hand right now, but by simply starting to deal with the issues and knowing you have a plan in place, it should stop these practical worries from using up your valuable headspace during the day.

2. Aim to take a pragmatic approach to any emotional worries (such as thinking you might have done a rubbish job or let someone down) by asking yourself whether you are thinking realistically. By being more objective you could find some of these worries are more to do with your perception than the real situation.

Is there any chance you could be:

- mental filtering – filtering out all the positives and only now seeing negatives;
- magnifying – enlarging the smallest negatives out of proportion;
- minimising – making the positives tiny;
- personalising – wrongly assuming you're to blame.

3. If you are plagued by an underlying anxious feeling, try thinking about where you were and what you were doing at the time you felt anxious. Over a few days, you should start to see a pattern emerging and, once you know the trigger to this anxious feeling, you can go back to the points above and start to deal with it. For example, you might find you feel a bit anxious and want to reach for a biscuit during meetings. Just pinpointing the trigger can be the first step to devising a plan to build confidence.

Quick fix

Stretch away the stress

When we're feeling stressed, it's easy for tension to build up in our bodies. This is because the stress response can cause muscle contractions – good for a short sprint to get away from danger, but not so good on a long-term basis. As a Scrambler you won't usually have the time to pop to a yoga or Pilates class every week, so try the hand stretching exercise opposite, that can be done anywhere.

Do as many or as few of hand stretches as you can throughout the day; you don't need to do the entire set – little and often is a more realistic approach for a Scrambler. But do try and top and tail with a few deep breaths each time you stretch so that you can destress as much as possible. Your kids and colleagues may even want to get involved! Hand stretches are also great for people who spend much of their time typing or doing other repetitive actions, and indeed can help with repetitive strain injury (RSI).

- Inhale through your nose for a count of three, feeling your belly rise, and exhale through your nose for three counts.

- Prayer stretch: First put your palms flat together in front of your chest as if you're praying, above the height of your chest. Now lower your hands towards your lap and you should feel the stretch in your fingers, palms and wrists. Hold this pose for a count of five before gently bringing your hands back up to parallel with the chest, and release. Repeat this exercise but now hold the stretch for a count of 10 before release.

- Stop finger stretch: Lift your right arm straight in front of you as if you were telling someone to 'stop'. Next, rotate your hand so that your fingers are facing the floor. Starting with your little finger, use your left hand to massage the finger from its base to the tip, then gently pull the finger towards your body for a stretch for a count of three. Do this with each finger, then switch to the left hand.

- Fisticuffs: Lift your arms in front of you again and make fists. First rotate your fists in circles towards each other for a count of 10, then in opposite directions for a count of 10. Repeat three times if possible.

- Shake it out: To end the exercise, put your arms at your sides shake your hands and wrists out for at least 10 counts. Finally, breathe in again for three counts and out for three, saying the word 'calm' in your mind.

Have a cup of tea

A simple cup of tea really can reduce stress. Researchers measured markers of stress and subjective feeling of stress in tea drinkers and non-tea drinkers[112] and found that tea drinkers are less stressed and more relaxed. So, if you're ever feeling a bit overwhelmed with your Scrambler life, take a couple of minutes for a cup of tea. If you already drink a lot of tea, consider swapping out a few cups for a herbal variety as too much caffeine throughout the day can lead to irritability and restlessness.

Do your homework
(slow-build, longer-term hacks)

Chase away your inner impostor

Even high achievers can harbour a constant, nagging fear that they'll be 'found out' as an impostor and this can lead to stress, anxiety and even depression.[113] 'Impostor Phenomenon' (also known as Impostor Syndrome), or the inability to truly accept that you are worthy of your accomplishments, affects men and women in all walks of life and across cultures. In fact, as many as 70% of people will experience Impostor Phenomenon at some stage in their lives.[114]

These feelings and behaviours can lead to procrastination or extreme over-preparation (two sides of a perfectionistic coin), then often frenzied preparation before a task. This is frankly exhausting and results in fatigue, burnout and poor habits such as erratic and unhealthy eating patterns. If you recognise this trait in yourself, you can work to free yourself from this phenomenon by trying these tips:

- Re-write your internal script. If you find yourself thinking something like, 'They should have hired someone else – I'm not good enough for this position,' then change your inner dialogue to something more positive like, 'I have a lot to offer in this role and was hired because I'm the right person for the job.'
- Talk it out. Share your feelings either with a trusted mentor or friend who might be better placed to separate reality from your insecurities.
- Change the angle. Scramblers often feel they are being judged on their performance but subtly shifting the expectation from 'performing' to 'teaching' effectively moves the focus on to others.

SHRINKOLOGY SCIENCE: IMPOSTOR PHENOMENON

Impostor Phenomenon was first conceived in 1978 by psychologists Pauline Clance and Suzanne Imes, who found a common combination of the following traits in people with high personal expectations:

- often succeed on tasks that they feared they'd do badly at;
- avoid evaluations as they fear negative feedback
- dismiss positive feedback as down to luck or other external circumstances
- fear that other people will discover the 'true' person who isn't as capable as others perceive them to be
- feel guilty or fearful when successful
- fear failure
- feel the need to be the very best or superhuman

- See it as a journey. All work, whether in an office or at home, is a journey. There are bumps along the way which help us learn from experience. By focusing less on the accomplishment and more on the process, the fear of being 'found out' might diminish.
- Tackle perfectionist tendencies. Use the Magpie's mind hacks on page 151.

By chasing away your inner impostor you'll feel less stressed in all the activities that a Scrambler throws into life.

Try setting healthier boundaries

Scramblers love to be busy and this can lead them to saying yes too often for their own good. Even though Scramblers like to do it all – and they can – they can find their boundaries are overly flexible.

Strict boundaries can be very useful when it comes to stress control. Establishing a clear boundary helps to clearly communicate your limits to others. It may seem counter-intuitive (especially to a Scrambler) but sometimes saying 'no' can heighten other's respect for you. Letting other people know how far they can push you is a great way for them to see your strengths more clearly.

It can be really quite surprising how people accept a line drawn in the sand. Fixed and stable boundaries help ease stress and benefit relationships immensely. We sometimes think our partners, friends, family and close colleagues should automatically know what we need, but remember that none of us are mind readers. No one will like you less for making things clear!

To start setting boundaries it's important to first look at where yours might be a bit 'wobbly'. Explore home, work, relationships and, in these areas, ask yourself if there are times when you feel over-whelmed, angry or frustrated? The need to be alone? Disrespected or taken advantage of?

INSTANT COURAGE BUILDERS

Bolster your courage with these psych hacks:

- Calm yourself first with a few minutes of slow deep breathing
- Use clear, unambiguous language like 'I need ... ', 'I will no longer ... ' (avoid saying 'you need' as it can make people defensive)
- Stick to your guns and follow through as this will increase others' respect for you
- Don't make excuses or apologise as this confuses the message
- If someone starts to push the boundary, don't hesitate to firmly, and calmly, point this out.

Now, once you know where the wobbly boundaries are, pick out the easiest one to push back on first. This could be something as simple as asking your partner to empty the dishwasher every other day. Once you've set and solidified one relatively straightforward boundary, move on to the next. The more you set, the easier the process becomes, and you will eventually be able to handle tricky boundaries with ease.

Scrambler's eat-less tips and tricks

Scramblers tend to be so busy rushing around achieving goals, keeping those plates spinning and making sure everyone else is happy and settled, that it is all too easy for your own diet and health concerns to drop further and further down your never-complete to-do list. You might be the go-to person for help but you Scramblers rarely spend time thinking about your own health or longevity.

You might think you eat virtually nothing and be utterly confounded by your weight gain, but one glimpse at your food/mood diary is very likely to reveal erratic eating behaviour and an unhealthy reliance on junk and convenience foods. This fast and furious approach to eating inevitably means compromise in terms of nutritional balance, which is certainly not sustainable or healthy, and it is not conducive to long-term weight maintenance. The tough truth is you are very likely to be the beating heart of your family or firm and you cannot expect your poor body and brain to cope with the relentless pressure you put it under, unless you put quality fuel into the tank.

- Structure your meals. **Weight maintenance for the Scrambler is all about injecting a little structure into eating patterns, and shifting the emphasis a little so your health creeps just a little higher up your never-ending to-do list by re-establishing a healthy rhythm with regular nutrition-packed meals. For you, the Shrinkology Fundamentals (Chapter 6) are crucial.**
- Sunday night is planning night. **Make sure you allocate one ring-fenced hour every Sunday evening to food planning and preparation for the week ahead. That doesn't mean making sure the kids have their favourite wrapped snacks for their lunch boxes, this is about you. Make the most of your methodical nature and run through your weekday plans to check there's time for a healthy sit-down meal either at lunchtime or early evening each day.**

Are there social engagements to be negotiated? Will you be forced to skip a meal or eat highly calorific food?

- Room to breathe. Sort out your own oxygen mask first each morning – no matter how insistent your mobile phone, or how many others are clamouring for your attention, try to stop for a moment and consider the practicalities of how you are going to get your properly nutritious main meal today. Does this mean whipping up a salad to take to work with you? Or taking something out of the freezer to defrost in time for supper? Just as you shouldn't be fiddling around with everyone else's oxygen masks while you're gasping for air in an in-flight emergency, you need to know that you'll be far more use to your dependants or colleagues if you've got yourself sorted first.

- Try two-for-one evening meals. If you've got into the very common habit of organising two meals each day – a late afternoon meal for the children and an early evening for the adults – consider combining the two. Children benefit enormously from being introduced to 'adult' meals – it's a great way to watch, listen and learn. Shared mealtimes are a very good opportunity to sit and properly connect in a relaxed manner. It cuts your meal prep time in half, and allows you to reap the benefits of eating your last meal of the day relatively early, effectively putting you in a shorter eating/longer fasting pattern. Perhaps brush your teeth afterwards to signal to your brain that there will be no more eating today.

- No picking. If your children are too young to eat adult food and need to eat separately, just make sure you've got cut-up vegetables on hand to nibble as you prepare, and if they leave tempting morsels of pickable bits on their plates, be ruthlessly efficient about scraping them into the bin, or keep a spray gun ready with a dilute solution of washing up liquid to spritz the leftovers and put you off completely.

- Snack mindfully. When we snack, we are especially prone to mindlessness so be alert to the seductive charms of the quick nibble. If you are tempted by a biscuit or a handful of peanuts try bringing your awareness to your body sensations, thoughts and emotions, and ask: Why am I eating this food? Am I bored? Am I actually hungry? If so, what's a healthy choice? What's going to make my body feel good?

- Turn your snacks into mini meals. If your life is so hectic you have to survive on snacks, shun the processed, shop-bought varieties and make sure your snacks are more like properly balanced 'mini meals' which balance protein (meat, fish, eggs, pulses), slow-burning carbohydrates (oat cakes, wholemeal bread), and healthy fat (nuts, seeds, avocado). Keep cut-up celery, carrots, sugar snap peas and other vegetables in the fridge (and at work if possible).

- Think French. If you have a tendency to live on air and black coffee all day, then find yourself unable to stop diving into a huge evening meal, try thinking French and add a salad course to every meal. Just make sure your fridge is well stocked with fresh, prepared salad (ok, you're a Scrambler, think bagged salad and cherry tomatoes instead) and sit down to a very large bowl of salad dressed in a deliciously piquant olive oil dressing with your evening meal. Not only will you be notching two or three portions of vegetables in one hit, plus a plethora of healthy nutrients, you should be able to slow the chaotic progress of your hunger hormones.

- Sit and go s-l-o-w. Make a pact with yourself to stop eating on the hop. Don't allow any food in your mouth unless you're sitting at the table, knife and fork in hand (napkin on your lap if you feel so inclined) with no phone, no radio, no TV, no newspaper, magazine or book. Instead, really, really focus on the food.

- Chew! Chew! Chew! Studies show more chewing equals less food.[115] Chew each mouthful of food (even soup, bizarrely) at 12 times to slow everything down and you'll end up eating less.

- Have a healthy breakfast. Although some Shrinkology types
  (notably Gourmets) might benefit from skipping the first meal
  in the day, a good breakfast is pretty important for the Scrambler.
  If you've got a chaotic day ahead, you don't have to add hunger
  and cravings into the mix. Aim to start your day with a healthy
  slow-burn breakfast even if you're not hungry (eggs are best)
  and you'll be more likely to make healthier food choices
  throughout the day.
- Stake out the office canteen. If your only lunchtime option
  is an unhealthy office canteen you do have options:
  petition (hard) for a salad bar;
  go 'low carb' at lunchtimes and fill your plate with protein
  (meat/fish) and vegetables;
  bring your own salad to work in a Kilner jar;
  consider skipping lunch completely if you're following a fasting plan.
- Perfect your 'express chef' skills. The lucrative ready meals industry
  has been designed to persuade you that a processed pouring sauce
  or 'pierce and ping' microwave meals are the quickest possible
  route to sustenance when time is tight. But with the right cookery
  book or YouTube channel you'll soon learn you can get a healthy
  meal on the table cooked from scratch in super-fast time. Skip past
  the processed food in the freezer cabinets and make your way to
  the dark outer corners. If you dig deep in larger supermarkets you'll
  find frozen chopped onions, crushed garlic, roasted vegetables,
  chopped peppers, mushrooms, grated cheese ... which mean you
  can create delicious homemade meals without sugars, sweeteners
  or preservatives in as much time as it takes to find the can opener.

SCRAMBLER SOCIAL MEDIA SOS

One great targeted way for Scramblers to loosen the destructive hold that social media might have over their lives is to make a pact to power down at set times of day. Start when the kids are young (this one is impossible to set up retrospectively with teenagers) and lead by example: place a special basket by the front door and ask that everyone, visitors included, places their phone in a basket when they walk in. At the very least, aim to set a few self-imposed limits: no phone at meal times; no phone two hours before bed; no phone when you're with people you love. Plus aim to use an alarm clock to wake you up in the morning rather than your phone, so that checking your feed is not the first thing you do before you greet each other each morning.

The Scrambler's diet digest

As a Scrambler you are likely to have tried plenty of diets over the years, but your hectic lifestyle makes it difficult to stick to any strict plan. You haven't got time to start health food shopping and you can swiftly build resentment at the fact that the 'clean eating' role models leave you feeling guilty for your apparently shoddy nutrition.

Scramblers respond best to rules rather than arbitrary nutritional trends (like low-carb or gluten-free). You tend to have a deep respect for traditions, which means a diet with proper procedure and set plans is more likely to be successful for you longer term. You haven't got the time and energy for lots of reading and research, so any instructions have to be sensible, concise and clear. For any diet plan to work at this stage of your life, speed and convenience are absolutely crucial.

You are more likely to be successful with any plan which switches one meal a day with a homemade juice as long as that meal replacement is healthy and filling. The drink is portable with the added Scrambler advantage of one less meal to worry about. That's why meal replacement plans like SlimFast and GoFigure (a more natural meal replacement alternative available online) and can be effective for Scramblers as an emergency fall-back.

Any plan which advocates short periods of fasting (such as Dr Xand van Tulleken's 'One meal a day' or Max Lowery's *The 2 Meal Day*) could be useful to help you plan your nutritional profile around fasting windows. Scramblers are used to feeling hungry, and a meal missed on purpose is a weight off the mind. That's why the 16:8 plan (see page 133) could be perfect for you. If you're rushing out of the house in the morning there's every chance you're skipping breakfast anyway, and bringing your evening meal forward to share with the children (as we advised on page 203) makes it very straightforward for you to eat within that recommended 8-hour window. You've just got to resist the urge for a nightcap. But do allow yourself leeway at weekends and special occasions.

If you can afford them, postal plans (such as Diet Chef and Body Chef) are a good short-term hit. These companies will send you a box of balanced calorie-counted food each day. This can be a good kick-start for Scramblers as they take out the planning stage and get you in the habit of eating proper meals.

It's worth investigating the 'Cheats and Eats' plan (Cheats & Eats: Lifestyle Programme by Jackie Wicks and Rob Hobson) which is a flexible way to nudge yourself into a healthy diet without having to worry about calories. Vegetables, pulses and nutrient-dense foods are 'eats' which can be eaten without restriction, but everything else counts as a 'cheat' and cheats are limited. It's a great plan for the Scrambler as there's only one thing to think about –keeping track of those cheats. There's even an app to keep the calculation for you.

Scrambler tips to cut back on the booze

The 'I deserve this', end-of-the-day large glass of wine is a classic Scrambler drink.

- Replace that rewarding glass of wine with something equally rewarding that you can ritualise, sit down and really enjoy, such as a set-timed 'off-loading' phonecall with a close relative or friend, an hour's peace with a newspaper or magazine, or one episode of your favourite soap or series.
- When out with friends and the only one not drinking, try to cut off the possibility that you might start to feel hard done by, or possibly even bored by the drunken ramblings by making it your quest to find out something new about a friend. The results will be your reward.
- If you find yourself in a bar with friends (or at the mercy of a drink-swilling partner) and you are offered a tempting drink, practise the art of responding like this: 'No thanks I don't **want** a drink right now.' Using the word **want** is much more powerful and effective than saying, 'No thanks 'I **can't** have one.' Studies show using the 'w' word means you could be twice as successful at resisting. That's because 'can't' implies you are denying yourself something desirable, but 'don't want' is empowering.[116]
- Get ahead of the game and squeeze in a pre-booked, early morning fitness class after a night when you know you are going to be socialising. Knowing it's in your diary, and knowing you've already paid for it, will give you one more reason to say no to the booze.
- Make a list of 'if–then' alternatives to help you come up with clever plans ahead of time to avoid drinking situations. So **if** ... my partner offers me a big glass of wine in the evening, **then** I'll make sure I've got chilled non-alcohol wine in the fridge instead.
- Collect pebbles in a jar – one for every drink you didn't have. Then cash them in at the end of the month (£1 per pebble) and buy yourself a non-food treat.

The Scrambler's tailored exercise prescription

If you're struggling to factor healthy eating into your super-busy life, the thought of adding regular exercise into the mix can seem an impossible hurdle to climb. But there are plenty of Scramble-proof ways and means.

The concept of High Intensity Interval Training could have been invented purely with the Scrambler in mind. It is a scientifically proven way of shoe-horning maximum fitness benefits into the shortest possible amount of time. Whether you're walking, swimming, cycling or jogging, you just have to push yourself very hard for as little as 20 seconds, ease off to catch your breath, then push yourself hard again. That's it.

It doesn't matter if you're running on the spot, doing push-ups, star jumps or burpees, the structure of the programme is the same: push yourself as hard as you can for 20 seconds and rest for 10 seconds. This is one set. Repeat eight times. Aim to make it a non-negotiable part of your day. Studies at McMaster University in Canada have shown you can get the same health benefits of nearly an hour of steady aerobic exercise with just a single minute of hard

---

ARE YOU TOO BUSY TO EXERCISE?

If you have a favourite TV show you watch regularly then perhaps you're not too busy to exercise, you could simply be **choosing** not to.

exercising. Even interval 'walking' appears to produce better health results than walking at a steady state pace. As long as you vary the intensity you'll still derive proportionally more benefit from your workout than if you take things slowly. In terms of exercise psychology, intervals keep you engaged, which makes the time feel like it's going even faster than it is.

It is very important to push yourself hard. HIIT should never be easy, but it's only four minutes, and as you get fitter, your recovery time should dramatically improve. Since HIIT – if you do it properly – is tough on the body, you'll burn more calories afterwards as the body repairs itself. One 2001 study found you burn nearly 100 calories more during the 24 hours after a HIIT session. That's 700 calories a week if you commit to those four minutes every morning.

No matter how chaotic or stressed your life is, it is almost impossible to be too busy for four minutes of exercise – and the impact on your metabolism and your health can be remarkable. If you really don't have time in your busy scrambling day for exercise, you can still inject a little movement and activity in there somehow. Just aim to do whatever it takes to incorporate more movement into your day and reduce the stagnating time spent sitting.

Get into the habit of standing up to take any phone call or, better still, walk whenever you talk. When friends suggest meeting for coffee, suggest a walk instead. If the weather is bad, window shopping at a large-covered shopping centre works just as well. Put a ban on using the car for short trips, do a few sit-ups before getting out of bed in the morning and squats when you are brushing your teeth.

If you have an exercise bike, drag it out of the garage and position it in front of the TV, or pick up a mini pedal exerciser (available online for about £20) to use under your desk, or in place of your footstool so you can get your legs going round when you'd be otherwise inactive. Set an alert on your phone to ping every hour to remind you to run through a series of simple squats (stand up from your chair and lower yourself repeatedly so your bottom almost touches the chair before standing again), stretches, or push-ups against the wall.

If you fear your exercise commitment is likely to waver, stick to mornings because research shows that this way you are more likely to make exercise a regular habit (less likely to skip because something comes up … or you can't be bothered) but, for health reasons, evening exercise allows you to destress from the day, and your joints and muscles will be more flexible so you should be less prone to injury.

WORK OUT WHILE YOU WORK

It really is worth investigating the possibility of a standing desk, or a treadmill desk. Take the stairs rather than the lift at every opportunity, never sit when you can stand, or stand when you can walk, or walk slowly when you can walk fast and swing your arms.

Ring fence some time every weekend to do something active with children or friends, whether it's Frisbee in the park, bike rides, tennis or swimming. You'll be healthier for it and you'll be instilling very healthy habits in the next generation of Shrinkologists as well as spending quality time with people you value.

TRY YIN YOGA

This is a slow-paced, deep-stretching style of yoga that is incredibly relaxing. Yoga has been shown to reduce stress and improve overall wellbeing[117,118] but instead of focusing on cardio or fluid movement, Yin is all about getting into the deep connective tissues of your body (fascia) and allowing your breath to permeate into the tight areas. The class focuses on passive, seated stretches that target the connective tissues in the hips, pelvis and lower spine. Poses are held for anywhere between one and 10 minutes. The aim is to increase flexibility and encourage a feeling of release and letting go. It is a great way to learn the basics of meditation and stilling the mind, and useful (though difficult) for athletic types who need to release tension in overworked joints; it is also good for those who need to relax.

Yin yoga is often used in programmes that deal with addictions, eating disorders, anxiety and deep pain or trauma. This slow pace urges you to really think about feelings, sensations and emotions. It's **not** about strength training and developing lean muscles, but if you're a Scrambler, that hour (or 90 minutes) on the mat is time very well spent.

Brief Scrambler summary

Scramblers will scramble – you probably can't see that you have any choice in the matter right now – so just aim to stay on top of stress by practising your personalised Shrinkology hacks. These will help beat cravings, and instil in you a renewed sense of control. Use as many Shrinkology short cuts as you can when it comes to food prep and exercise and aim to carve out a little 'me' time into every day.

If you do just one thing ...

Just say 'no'. When you feel the stress rise up and know you're taking on too much, push back a little. You'll be amazed how others are totally capable of doing things they once unloaded onto you.

Chapter 12
The Soother

Who is The Soother?

The Soother is the best of friends. That's because Soothers have a genuine interest in others and spend a great deal of time and energy observing the likes and dislikes of the people you love, colleagues and friends – you buy the most thoughtful gifts. You take your responsibilities to heart and you are a dependable worker. But as you find it difficult to say 'no', you can become over-burdened, a common source of misery and stress that can lead you to search for solace in food.

Soothers tend to be intuitive and you like to use this insight to help others if you can. You'll be the first to spot the wallflower at a party, possibly because you know how that feels yourself. Not many people would guess this, but you're actually probably quite shy inside. As a child, some of your relatives might have been critical of your natural reticence and introversion, and tried to help by bringing you out of your shell even though you felt quite content playing on your own. Often sweet treats were used for this and also to soothe away tears or as a prize for good behaviour, so it seems completely natural to eat away any strong feelings. Because you care so much for others, you can't stand the thought that you might have hurt someone's feelings. You're a sensitive soul and you keenly feel other people's pain so you'll put a great deal of effort into making sure this doesn't happen. It's an admirable trait, but it can mean you end up ignoring your own needs, and in caring so much for others you might find any negative emotions of your own can be channelled inwards and masked with eating food.

Soothers tend to prefer structured environments and value security. You like to feel in control, so you generally follow the rules and don't let things get out of hand. Making other people happy is important to you and although you wouldn't miss a birthday party, wedding or christening you are very likely to be self-nominated designated driver, looking after the over-inebriated rather than really letting yourself go. You're not the sort to judge someone harshly for overstepping the mark, as you're more inclined to seek out reasons for someone's self-destructive behaviours and help them to overcome these.

You are likely to be deeply self-conscious about your weight, but your approach can swing between apparent self-confidence (big is beautiful, 'I'm happy as I am', more cuddly this way) and self-loathing. Not that anyone would know this. Food and your body shape are very personal issues for you. This is why friends and family might be surprised to know you struggle with your weight. They might think you are quite happy as you really *hate* anyone to be worrying about you, which makes it hard for you to ask for support.

Classic Soother eating behaviours

The Soother loves food, always has done, always will. Eating puts you in a kind of pleasure trance, and you just can't help yourself loving pasta and risotto, mash, chips and stodge, bread and toast at every opportunity – for you courgetti or cauliflower rice are just pretenders to the deliciously stodgy carbohydrate throne.

- Sweet tooth. You glean comfort and joy from puddings and desserts.
- You're a chocaholic. The brown stuff isn't optional. It is compulsory, every day.
- Eating emotionally. Because you were brought up to believe – even subconsciously – that food provides some kind of comfort when you are unhappy, bored or distressed, you can be vulnerable to a powerful psychological and physiological dependence on carbohydrates and sugar (see Chapter 1). You might be more inclined than most to eat in response to stress or anxiety, depression, loneliness or sadness, anger and frustration. For you, feeling any form of emotional distress can easily lead to an overwhelming desire to eat carb-laden foods to such an extent that you very often eat with almost no awareness. When this happens you can act like a sleepwalker working your way methodically through an entire box of chocolates. It feels great at first, but as the empty wrappers pile up, feelings of self-recrimination mount in equal proportion.
- Behind closed doors. It's when the Soother is alone that the overeating can be a problem. Many Soothers feel an element of shame about their secret eating habits. Carb-frenzied eating often happens alone, which in itself exacerbates the deep-seated feelings of low worth. You might try to kid yourself it doesn't matter what you eat because you're 'weak' and 'not worth cherishing'.
- Strong cravings. Our carb addiction will probably drive strong cravings, making it even more difficult than normal to choose healthy foods – even when low-carb and healthier foods are on offer, you're likely to opt for a sandwich (followed by a muffin or chocolate bar) instead of a more energy-balanced salad.
- Mindless eating. Because food can be used to mask any uncomfortable feelings, including boredom, the Soother is prone to mindless eating in front of the TV or on long journeys.

- Netflix and nibble. Escapism is one coping strategy very typical of Soother, so a box set of favourite shows will very often come as a neatly tied up package with a large bag of tortilla chips or a pack of Minstrels, which means a substantial calorie intake.
- Sharing is caring. As a Soother you like to feed others. You are probably an expert baker (or at the very least you know where to buy the best possible cakes), you put a great deal of time and effort into cake-making or selection, and there is always something lovely (and highly calorific) to eat when people come to visit your home. You are likely to be the 'office feeder' bringing in cakes for birthdays and the first to suggest a celebratory drink or lunch – not because you consciously want to eat, but because that seems like a lovely, warm, inclusive thing to do.
- You can't resist the treats drawer. You'll have a one of these in your kitchen (which means temptation is never far from your reach).
- Always hungry, never full. Sometimes you wonder whether you're missing whatever chemical messaging system other people have to signal fullness, because you can eat and eat and eat, until you are uncomfortably full, then, when everyone else has finished, find room for a dessert.
- In a hurry. You often eat fast. Really fast. Especially if you're hungry, 'hangry', or in a rush. You'll happily munch away while talking, walking, typing, and always taking great big mouthfuls and polishing off the lot super-fast.

Soother case study

Amy works as the deputy manager of a nursery in a small town where she lives with her boyfriend Eddie. Amy loves her job but is feeling increasing pressure from her boss and is taking on more responsibility (though no rise in wage). Eddie and Amy have a good relationship but it's under pressure from the nursery and the fact that they would like to start a family, but the time never seems right – because of other family commitments (ageing parents), not enough money, not in the right house/area, etc. This creates a deep sense of longing in Amy, even though she tells Eddie it's fine, they have plenty of time.

Childhood definitely felt like a magical time for Amy and she would love nothing more than to recreate this – everyone was happy and she felt safe and secure in her family home. Each scratched knee and bumped head was erased with a biscuit or snack – but feelings were never really discussed. Amy definitely doesn't recall even once seeing her dad cry, as men were men, and mums could soothe away anything unpleasant.

Amy notices chocolate wrappers stuffed in her car's glove compartment – sometimes she barely even remembers eating them at all and is a little surprised to find them there. This brings about a sense of shame that must be pushed down again – often with more food.

Eddie can sense that Amy is becoming distant, fading into herself, and tries to cheer her up by suggesting they go out. This seems like a wonderful idea at first and Amy shows enormous self-restraint by ordering the healthy salmon and steamed veg – but after pinching one of Eddie's chips things start to slide as she helps him finish them off. The stodgy sticky toffee pudding that follows leaves Amy almost euphoric – but this ecstasy soon wears off when they're home and she feels remorse. There certainly won't be any baby-making tonight …

The Soother's mind hacks

Mind hacks for the Soother focus on finding non-food sources of comfort and learning to develop an internal voice that can act as a supportive guide. For many Soothers it can be useful to look at the past as a way of helping you acknowledge and release any negative feelings. It is also useful to shift focus from food as a way of showing love and affection – even though this may be a behaviour you've learned in childhood and thus is very well-established, you DO have the power to make changes now to shape your future. Self-compassion is key for Soothers, so your hacks here will show you that you have to care for yourself as you would others.

DAILY HACKS

Affirm yourself – supportive self-talk

As Buddha (apparently) said: 'We are shaped by our thoughts; we become what we think.' While this may at first appear a little flaky, the scientifically backed principle of cognitive behaviour therapy (CBT; see page 172) is based on the idea that our thoughts influence our lives through their interaction with our behaviour – in other words we do indeed act out what we think.

If you genuinely think you are overweight, unattractive and unlovable you are probably less likely to go out, have fun and meet new people. But conversely, by simply telling yourself good things about your body, mind and relationships you can start to change how your feel and act – both towards yourself and others (see page 149). The activity over the page outlines how to introduce these hacks into your daily life.

SELF SUPPORT

Try writing a series of relevant affirmations about you that are positive, supporting sentiments. Think about the loveliest thing someone has said to you based on your numerous qualities or the nicest thing you'd love to say to a close friend, then phrase this in a self-statement such as:

- Body: 'I am full of energy and my body feels strong and ready for the day.'
- Mind: 'I have overcome many difficulties in the past and have the ability to conquer my challenges today.'
- Intellect: 'I am a clever individual and can use other ways to fill myself with knowledge and understanding instead of food.'
- Relationships: 'Because I respect myself I surround myself with people that support me.'

Affirmations can also be more specific, such as in the case of Amy:

- Body: 'I am strong and feel ready and able to take on my day at the nursery.'
- Mind: 'I am a good and compassionate person who makes people feel loved and cared for – including myself.'
- Intellect: 'I can use other ways to tackle cravings, such as engrossing myself in the hobbies I love.'
- Relationships: 'I have a deep and meaningful relationship with my partner that is based on trust and respect.'

At the start of each week, write down one affirmation in each category (body, mind, intellect, relationships), then, every day, stand in front of a mirror and read them out to yourself. It may feel odd at first, but stick with it. Self-affirmations help to buffer against stress and improve self-esteem by reminding us of our vast array of internal resources.[119] Also, by continually telling yourself these positive statements you'll be able to make new neural connections (see page 148) so that in time your mind will follow this new path that is hopeful, empowered and able to meet challenges head on without turning to food for comfort.

Crisis control for cravings

Put together a Hygge emergency box

Take a leaf out of our Scandinavian friends' book and make a box full of soothing objects. Hygge, which loosely means a 'sense of cosiness and comfort', can engender deep feelings of contentedness. Create your own Hygge supply by gathering together items such as:

- thick cosy bed socks;
- super-soft blankets;
- a delicious selection of exotic herbal teas;
- earthy scented candles and tea lights;
- beautiful natural objects like pinecones, twigs and colourful leaves that help you connect with nature.

Keep this box ready and whenever you fear you are about to be overwhelmed by cravings, take out its contents and immerse yourself in Scandi comfort.

Have a little weep

Sometimes a good sobbing session can leave you feeling better. 'Crying' is a known psychophysiological reaction made by many animals to pain or anger, characterised by howling, ranting and wailing – without tears. 'Weeping', however, is when we shed tears – and only humans do this. Scientists have found physiological differences between crying and weeping, in other words whether we shed tears or not. When we cry (without tears) our heart rate and blood pressure increase, adrenaline is produced and muscle and voice tone change (which allows animals to vocalise loudly). This explains how shouting can sometimes leave us feeling 'pumped'. The action of weeping (with tears), produces mood-soothing endorphins. The sensation of tears gently rolling down our face sends a calming massage to the brain. The tender rhythm of a sob is also thought to aid emotional relief and act as a comfort blanket. Weeping behaviours appear to trigger 'mirror neurons' in the brain which are responsible for our feelings of empathy. This means weeping isn't always a negative indication of weakness or ineptitude. It can be a very positive sign and a useful exercise which really can help us deal with sorrow or sadness.[120] So when you need a craving crisis fix, watch a heart-warming movie and don't hold back from letting the tears fall.

When you're alone

Calorie-free giving

Soothers love to give, but it might be useful to focus some of those well-meant 'giving' skills outside of food. A considerable amount of concentration and commitment needs to be channelled into craft-making, writing or growing plants, and the sense of accomplishment and wellbeing can, over time, help to replace the need to soothe with food (and will certainly give just as much joy to the recipient).

We all appreciate a handmade or personalised gift, and because you are very unlikely to be the only one in your social circle that is watching their weight, non-food gifts are likely to be gratefully received.

Keeping yourself occupied and your fingers busy will also restrict your opportunities for mindless eating. Try:

- Complex knitting or crochet – ditch the boring old scarf patterns and crochet animals and search for challenging patterns online (Pinterest is a great source of inspiration). If you'd rather stick to big projects like quilts, research the charities that support premature baby units, cancer wards and others in hospitals, giving your efforts to a truly good cause.
- Jewellery making – add an intimate twist by asking friend if they a have a single earring or a broken piece that you could turn into something new
- Up-cycling – you don't need to be a master carpenter to breathe fresh life into an old piece of furniture. Start with online tutorials and get creative!

Quick fix

Soothe with massage

A massage shouldn't be thought of as a frivolous luxury, only for birthdays and special occasions. Research has shown that hands-on treatments have important therapeutic and biochemical effects on our bodies.[121] Massage therapy also helps in a host of medical conditions, including prenatal depression, autism, skin problems, pain syndromes including arthritis and fibromyalgia, high blood pressure, autoimmune conditions including asthma and multiple sclerosis, HIV, breast cancer and neurodegenerative problems including Parkinson's and dementia.[122] One reason that people benefit from massage is that it increases levels of serotonin (the 'happy' hormone) by as much as 28 per cent and reduces cortisol (the 'stress' hormone) by as much as 31 per cent.

You may still want to book yourself a glorious pamper day but this isn't usually something that can act as a quick fix. So when you face a strong craving for chocolate and you suspect you are chasing a feel-good fix, try giving yourself a quick face massage instead. It is a completely calorie-free exercise with longer lasting impact than the 3-minute boost you might get from chocolate.

Ground control to Major Tom

Who doesn't want to be an astronaut and feel weightless? Instead of studying and training for years, use your own bathroom to experience weightlessness and a sense of space travel. We all have the ability to free ourselves from our physical bodies – as long as there's a bath! To prepare a mind-freeing bath, simply:

- Fill the bath with water to a temperature comfortable to you.
- Turn down the lights or fill the room with candles.
- Add 2 cups of Epsom salts to the water – adding salt to water changes its density so you'll feel more buoyant. This is why we can float more easily in the sea or ocean compared to a freshwater lake.
- Wear earplugs to block out any external sound.
- You may want to set a timer as it can be hard to know how much time has passed when you're liberated from external stimulation.

Now all you'll hear is the sound of your beating heart. If any thoughts enter your mind, acknowledge them as 'thoughts' as you would in a mindfulness exercise, and nudge them back into space.

Massage therapy

First, either use your favourite brand of face oil or serum, or you
can make one yourself: to a teaspoon of base oil (e.g. apricot kernel
oil for dry or mature skin; camellia or jojoba for all skin types;
grapeseed oil for oily skin), add a couple of drops of essential oils
(e.g. orange blossom or sandalwood for dry or mature skin;
grapefruit and tea tree for acne and breakout-prone skin; lavender
for combination or sensitive skin).*

1. Warm up: warm up your fingers first with hot water to help
distribute the oils and increase blood flow.
2. Chin up: now, use your fingers and palm in upwards, smooth
but slow sweeping movements on both sides of the face for
an invigorating massage (x 5). For a more relaxing technique,
move the hands back down once you reach your forehead (x3).
3. Forehead tension ease: now place both sets of fingertips
(index, middle and ring fingers) in the centre of your forehead.
Apply some comfortable pressure here and draw the fingertips
out to the sides of the face (x3).
4. Eye-soothe: the skin around the eyes is very delicate (hence this is
the area where fatigue can show) so go lightly on the amount of oil
here and the pressure. Start by placing your index and middle fingers at
the sides of your face, just where your eyebrows stop. In small, circular
motions, very gently work around the eye socket, up the bridge of
the nose, then over the eyebrows back to the starting point (x1).
5. Cheek circles: use circular motions again for this last technique.
Start at the top of your cheekbone near your temples and use the
length of the index and middle fingers to make firmer, rounded
movements. Steadily move down to below the cheekbone, next to
the ear. Then move slightly back up and along the cheekbone (x2).

* If you have any allergies do make sure you can tolerate the oils by first doing a small patch test.

Do your homework
(slow-build, longer-term hacks)

Putting the past to bed

This exercise will help you to process difficult past experiences which might be unconsciously creeping in to your relationship with food. Take out your journal, paper and pen, or even type on a device if you prefer. Start to write down the situation that was distressing – this may be difficult and some powerful emotions may rise to the surface. If this happens, practise deep breathing (see page 189) and try to sit with the memory, rather than pushing it away (or feeding it with negative thoughts). Write this as a short story with a clear beginning, middle and end – you needn't become lost in the fine detail here. Now, take a moment before reading the story and ask yourself:

- **WHAT ARE THE OBJECTIVE FACTS IN THIS STORY?** Focus on the tangible events in the story including the age of the narrator and the environment.
- **WHAT ARE THE EMOTIONS, PERCEPTIONS AND JUDGEMENTS CLOUDING THE OBJECTIVE FACTS HERE?**
- **WHY AM I HOLDING ONTO THIS MEMORY?** (E.g. I'm scared of letting it go as I might make the same mistake again/open myself to feeling this way again in the future, etc.)

Take your time with this. Now check in with yourself and ask if you're ready to let this memory go. If the answer is no, that's ok – this is a powerful exercise. You can gently start to use emotional writing practices by noting down daily experiences as this helps to process thoughts and feelings too. When doing both types of expressive writing, however, make sure to place yourself in the picture by using pronouns (e.g. I, me, myself) as this helps us to think about and come to terms with events and our relationship with others.[123]

Sunny side up

Another very easy way to boost serotonin levels is with sunlight.[124] Take a 20-minute walk, even if it's overcast, as you'll still soak-up natural light. If this isn't possible, invest in a light box or natural light alarm clock. These clocks gradually emit light to replicate the rising sun, which can make it easy to wake in the morning and help banish seasonal blues.[125] There are also desk lamp versions of light boxes if you spend a lot of time doing office work.

How to have your cake – and eat it mindfully

Mindless eating is one big reason diets so rarely seem to work, but mindfulness can help break those 'mindless' food associations and nibbling habits you might have got into over the years. Practising a few simple mindfulness techniques every day will help you build your self-awareness with the aim that you should be able to nudge yourself out of autopilot and think clearly about what you are about to put in your mouth.

Mindfulness works in many ways to help us be less reactive to food information, and so less likely to eat unthinkingly. It also gives our satiety signals time to tell us we're full.

Don't think of cake as banned, but if you do indulge, enjoy and appreciate it very slowly. Normally, the pleasure we receive from any food will build, peak (at a point called 'taste satiety' which should trigger a shift in the brain), and then start to decline. The point we reach taste satiety will depend on the size of the bites we take, how hungry we were when we started eating, the speed at which we eat, whether we're eating whole or processed food, and the flavour mix in the food. When it's working normally, our taste satiety mechanism tells us we've 'had enough' of that particular flavour, but the message will be subtle, and you have to slow down and pay attention to hear it. Most Soothers will have to listen very, very hard. Try this trick to train the fine-tuning of your satiety mechanisms:

1. Put a small slice of chocolate cake in front of you, close your eyes and breathe deeply for a few seconds.

2. Open your eyes and pick up the plate. Take a really good look at that piece of cake, noticing the size, shape, colours and textures. Inhale deeply – what flavours can you smell?

3. Slowly cut the cake into tiny bite-sized pieces and put a piece on your tongue, but do not bite it. What do you now notice about the flavour? Move it around your mouth. Does it taste different in different parts of your mouth? Allow it to melt on your tongue. What do you notice as it melts?

4. Take as long as you like to chew and eat the cake. Can you feel it move out of your mouth, into your throat? Into your stomach? Be aware of any thoughts or emotions that pass through, distinguishing them from a sensation like taste.

5. Continue eating the cake very slowly, one piece at a time, putting your fork down between mouthfuls and really noticing how the flavours blend in your mouth. That cake has the same number of calories whether eaten in three bites or 15, but the satisfaction you get from it can be so much more intense.

6. Take time over each bite, and ask yourself repeatedly if you've had enough. When you have had enough, stop. By slowing down like this you're likely to feel satisfied more quickly and stop earlier, or at least refuse a second slice.

A present to yourself – be present

Soothers can use food to help them feel good but there are other, more mindful, ways to self-care. Mindful self-compassion practice is a good way to give yourself a gift – not a fleeting token that's 'a moment on the lips, a lifetime on the hips', but rather a long-lasting and fundamentally life-changing daily present to yourself. In Buddhism, the term 'metta' means a sense of love (platonic rather than romantic), kindness, good-will, benevolence and amity towards others. As a Soother this will be second nature to you, but the question is, how can you redirect these feelings towards yourself?

For Soothers self-compassion doesn't come naturally – while you are excellent at making others feel warm inside and cared for, these skills are not often used on yourself. This isn't surprising as self-compassion takes conscious effort and practice –but you can use the great deal of expertise you've accumulated in taking care of others for yourself in this TLC exercise.

1. Start with simply noticing yourself. Be aware of your presence – allow your mind to tune into your physical sensations, starting with your breath. You don't need to do any special breathing exercises here, simply notice how it feels to breathe, either with your eyes open or closed. Explore this sensation with curiosity and non-judgement. Then scan your body for any other sensations such as heaviness and tension.

2. Think about someone you care deeply for. Gently gather and softly knead together the feelings of metta, i.e. compassion, love, warmth, kindness and care you feel towards this person in a mental hug.

3. Focus your thoughts. Home in on the following statements:

a. May _____ (add name) feel a sense of happiness and freedom in their life.

b. May _____ experience a sense of calm, harmony and serenity in their life.

c. May _____ find their inner strength to cope with the challenges that face them.

d. May _____ experience a lessening in their personal suffering.

4. Check in with your bodily sensations. How does this feel? What physical sensations do you notice now? Perhaps your breathing has slowed down; perhaps the tension in your shoulders has diminished; perhaps you feel somewhat lighter. You may even be smiling.

5. Focus your mind's eye on the images you can see when thinking of this person. Can you see them feeling happy and joyous? Again, approach this with curiosity and an open mind.

6. Try to refocus these thoughts onto yourself – put yourself in the place of your loved one. Say to yourself (it needn't be aloud):

a. May I feel a sense of happiness and freedom in my life.

b. May I experience a sense of calm, harmony and serenity in my life.

c. May I find their inner strength to cope with the challenges that face me.

d. May I experience a lessening in my personal suffering.

7. End the session by bringing your awareness back to your breath. Focus on the inhale and exhale for a few moments before ending the exercise.

Soother's eat-less tips and tricks

Soothers tend to have a complex and often unhealthy relationship with food. You might look on in wonder at friends who eat when they are hungry and stop when they are full. For you, food is so much more than mere sustenance. As a first step, it is really important for you to read, analyse and absorb the Shrinkology Fundamentals in Chapter 6.

You probably find it difficult *not* to eat sweet and stodgy foods if they are easily within reach, so your kitchen needs to be especially clear and virtuous, and packed with healthy options. Putting any barrier (like using a foil wrapping rather than cling film on left-overs) will help slow your propensity for mindless grazing.

- Know your rewards. Check your food/mood diary for your food consumption habits. Now make a separate note of all the potential 'rewards' that might be driving your eating or drinking loop. Is it social interaction that you crave? Stress relief? Boredom relief? Make a list of alternative suggestions that give you the same rewards (a breathing exercise, affirmation exercise, do an exercise class or go to the coffee shop).
- Understand your unhelpful eating habits. Go through your diary and pick out your most unhelpful eating habits . Do you always order a muffin with your latte? Does queuing to pay for fuel also mean buying a chocolate bar? Does your lap feel empty without popcorn when you're at the movies? The key to breaking an unhelpful habit is to pinpoint your trigger (a certain mood, a time of day, or a specific ritual) and insert a non-food ritual in its place.
- Get ready to graze, on your terms. Before you go to bed every evening, make fill a sealed container with crudités (such as carrots, cucumber, pepper, celery, mini cherry tomatoes) on which you can graze happily through the following day.

- Are you really hungry? Before you put anything in your mouth, stop and ask yourself: Why am I eating this? Is this food supporting my health? How will I decide when to stop eating? Will a couple of bites be enough? Every time you feel an urge to eat, ask yourself, 'What do I really need right now?' You may be surprised by the answer – do you really need food, or does your body need a break? A glass of water? A hug?

- Mini treats. Soothers can come unstuck if there is no sweetness in their lives, so keep a store of mini treats that enable you to satisfy a craving without ruining all your best weight-loss intentions. Ensure all your dessert 'treats' are frozen ones, so you can whip something out and defrost it speedily if needed. If you *must* have biscuits and crisps, store them out of sight and out of reach (in the garage or the attic?) because any effort required in accessing them should be enough to jolt you out of the mindless eating model.

- No more guilt. If you decide to say yes to the slice of cake, make sure you really, really enjoy it. Make every mouthful count. Don't allow yourself to feel guilty. If you do it, do it properly or don't do it at all.

- Snap out of it: If you're the sort to wander around the kitchen in a trance, picking bits off the children's plates, or breaking biscuits in half (and then going back for the other half) try wearing an elastic hair band around your wrist. As you feel the urge to reach into the biscuit tin, ping the band. It won't hurt, but the sharp sensation will send a mild 'pain' message to your brain which makes a tenuous link between biscuits and pain. Repeat the process often enough and you'll form a neural pathway which will bring grazing out of the depths of your subconscious into a more considered and more easily controlled behaviour. In studies, researchers gave drinkers a mild electric shock when they reached for a drink and observed that eventually they found the idea of alcohol repugnant.[126] This form of 'aversion therapy' can work because it puts a negative association (the sharp pain of the elastic band) in your brain alongside the urge, so subconsciously you start to associate the thought of that item of food or drink with an unpleasant sensation. Certainly the ping brings the thought of eating or drinking into the conscious mind, so you are less likely to act mindlessly, and more likely to at least think twice.

- Slow down your eating. Halve the pace. Start each meal with a few moments of conscious awareness, take your first mouthful, then put your knife and fork down and really enjoy what you are tasting before diving in for another mouthful. Stop your meal after ten bites and check your hunger and fullness signals.

- Phone a friend. Find a 'diet buddy' with similar weight-loss aspirations as yours. Soothers love to support others and you will certainly benefit from the encouragement. Studies show your chances of success are increased if you tell others about your quest (you are less likely to want to let each other down) and the growing friendship will boost your feelings of self-worth and reduce your risk of emotional eating.

- Turn down the volume dial on your carbohydrate consumption. If you stick close to your Shrinkology Fundamentals, you will be filling at least half your plate with vegetables, and protein (meat, fish, eggs or pulses) are a very important part of every meal to help maintain muscle and keep you feeling fuller for longer. So, instead of building a veritable volcano of carbohydrate and placing meat and veg on top, get used to just putting a large spoonful on the side.

- Control your sugar addiction. Soothers are the most likely Shrinkology type to be sugar addicts. Your love of sweet things can set you on a rollercoaster of blood sugar highs and lows and impossible-to-resist cravings for more, more, more. Possibly the single most important move you could make is to cut back on sugar. Start with the white stuff – sugar in coffee, tea and sprinkled on cereal. Then reduce your consumption of desserts and 'treats'. Use a smaller spoon for sugar in tea or coffee, and mix 'no sugar added' cereal 50:50 if the household has a high-sugar favourite. If you bake at home, use slightly less sugar. Try swapping syrup or honey on yoghurt or porridge for berries (fresh or frozen), and switching biscuits for oatcakes. You'll notice the cravings diminish and gradually your taste buds will sharpen to the point where savoury foods start to taste sweet. Stealth sugar-reduction works – a study in the *American Journal of Clinical Nutrition* found that after two months on a lower-sugar diet, participants perceived sugary foods to be 40 per cent sweeter than before.[127]

• Reward yourself for beating cravings. Put a piece of dried pasta in a jar for every time you beat a craving, and take a piece of pasta out every time you succumb. When the jar is full, treat yourself to a massage, or sitting down to read a chapter of your book.

Soother social media SOS

As a Soother your social media feed is more likely to be made up of old friends dating back to childhood as you love to stay in touch, even if it is just a voyeuristic connection. But sometimes the pixie dust of social media can make other people's lives seem impossibly perfect, and when you're feeling down, a finger flick through various school friends' glamorous summer holiday snaps can sour even the most positive mood and lead you to seek solace in the contents of the fridge.

You know you only post your most flattering photos and delete or hide any that show imperfections, but it is all too easy to forget that this is what everyone else is doing too! Time for a reality check. Your little cousins might look cherubic on that sun-kissed beach, but there's every chance they were a complete nightmare throughout the entire flight getting there.

The antidote to any inevitable resentment you might feel building is to stop watching and actually connect with some of your social media 'friends'. Once you can properly interact with them you'll get so much more out of the relationship and no doubt come to realise that the apparent perfection we all portray is a very flimsy fragile façade. We are all paddling furiously underneath!

You can also investigate different ways to make your love of social media work to help your weight loss journey rather than hold you back or embitter you. Try searching for support groups online. A Northwestern US University found that online dieters who checked into CalorieKing, a weight-loss website, to log their meals and 'friend' other dieting members, lost 8 percent more body weight after six months than their less-connected peers.[128]

One clever way to give yourself a positive uplifting boost multiple times a day is to change your computer password to something which could help you reach your goals. Since we all use passwords a lot, a positive, helpful, uplifting password could filter positive thoughts into your life, which could help you stay on track with your healthy eating. Try your own clever combinations – something like 1eat@ well or happy@me.

This practice, salted nicely throughout the day, might counterbalance the tendency to experience negative emotions or unhelpful thoughts which can lead to disordered eating. To be really effective, your passwords should state what you plan to do, and not use negatives, so 'ismilealot' will work better than 'idonotfrown'.

Tip: change your password regularly (at least every month) to keep up with your changing goals and try to add codes or symbols so it isn't too easy to crack.

The Soother's diet digest

The most common mistake Soothers tend to make is to pick a low-carb diet plan. You know carbohydrates are your downfall and you not surprisingly believe that cutting out carbs will be your best possible route to everlasting slenderness. You'll probably have tried Atkins (low-carb high-fat), and dabbled with Dukan (low-carb, low-fat) with a degree of success. Initially.

You are very likely to have benefitted from better blood sugar control (which is a very good thing) and you will have had to be very mindful of what you could and couldn't eat. You will also have been sailing on the hurricane force of enthusiasm, determination and the rapidly descending numbers on the scales as your body burnt up the glycogen stores in your tissues and you shed the water that is normally stored alongside it.

But carb-free living can be very difficult long term and for the Soother it can swiftly seem like a life sentence ('no fluffy mashed potato in my life for ever and ever?!?'). More than any other Shrinkology type, the Soother will always and inevitably be lured back by the temptation of the squidgy inside of a baguette or the crinkle cut chip on someone else's plate.

The Shrinkology Solution is not about denial, deprivation or making things any harder for you than they have to be. Be honest with yourself: you are never going to want to tolerate life long term without a carb-crutch, but you can reduce emotional reliance on carbs, turn the spotlight down, and nudge gently towards a healthier approach to food.

Soothers are better advised to choosing a long-term eating plan that allows carbs but gradually reduces dependence and makes them more complex (wholegrain), to calm cravings, reduce insulin resistance and get back in control.

So when looking for a diet, investigate structured plans that allow carbs and treats in moderation. The Shrinkology message is all about the long term, and being honest. You're not going to stick at any plan long term if it denies you chocolate, chips or bread.

For Soothers, organised groups like Weight Watchers and Slimming World might work well because they foster a spirit of teamwork and support which studies have shown can help. Of all the Shrinkology types, this helps the Soother most.

Meal replacement diets and the whole juice/smoothie genre are less likely to be successful because many Soothers hate to feel excluded or 'on a diet'. Soothers also prefer a structured environment and strict rules, so don't expect instant success from a regime that advocates sticking to broad dietary principles (the Mediterranean diet) or which proudly proclaims 'no calorie counting or portion control required' (alkaline diet or 'clean eating'). You're likely to see more success if your food and your progress are measured.

Aim to find a structured three-meals-a-day plan which heroes carbohydrates and allows occasional snacks and clever no-sugar desserts. If you can afford a 'delivered-to-your-door' diet plan for a few weeks, it can be a useful way to train your body and brain to expect new healthier foods and smaller portions. But aim to wean yourself off the plan and back on to your own two nutritionally healthy feet.

Many Soothers are self-confessed sugar-fiends but if you've lived a life of carbohydrate-based meals you could be at greater risk of type 2 diabetes. If your doctor has warned you that this is the case, you might see great success with Dr Michael Mosley's Blood Sugar Diet. It offers three options: a fast and furious kick-start on 800 calories a day; a 5:2 version whereby you eat 800 calories a day for two days and a special healthy diet for the rest of the week; and a low-carb, Mediterranean-style diet for longer term weight maintenance. You can follow the plan by reading his book (The Blood Sugar Diet, published by Short Books) or join one of his 12-week online programs (see www.thebloodsugardiet.com).

Soother tips to cut back on the booze

Pouring yourself a stiff G&T to cheer yourself up, or a cosy Netflix and chill-night with friends, wine and comfort food is second nature to a Soother. Here's how to kick the habit for good.

- If most of your drinking is done at home, take steps to remove temptation by emptying your old drinks cabinet. Remove whatever you have – even the old dregs of Amaretto might suddenly seem very appealing when a big craving strikes – and re-stock the fridge and cupboards with alcohol-free alternatives. Have the bottom tray in your fridge stashed with temptingly chilled no-alcohol beer and wine to offer as an option when friends come over.
- The Soother loves to help others, so consider a sponsored month of sobriety – it's a great way to strengthen your resilience, prove that you CAN do it, and put money into a worthy cause at the same time.
- Whizz up a deliciously indulgent hot chocolate instead. It might be 160 calories, which might seem excessively indulgent if you've been on (and off) a diet for most of your life but it's considerably less than the 250 cals in a large glass of wine and you're much less likely to open a packet of crisps or peanuts to go with it, pour yourself a second glass (another 250 cals) or wake up feeling ropey the next morning and craving a sugar-packed breakfast.
- When you really, really fancy a drink, think happy thoughts instead. Studies at Canada's McGill University found thinking about the place you were happiest works better at cravings control than trying to distract yourself with mathematical equations because it delivers a positive burst of reward.

The Soother's tailored exercise prescription

The best form of activity for the Soother is fun and sociable – a get-together with friends where you get a bit puffed, stretched out or pumped up muscles. At the very least, find a walking friend and dog-walk together every day, or gather three other friends to play doubles tennis with – no matter how many excuses your subconscious comes up with, you're going to struggle to bail because it means letting the others down. Group fitness classes suit you best, especially if they are fun and energetic.

EXERCISE TO REDUCE CRAVINGS

Regular exercise is the dieter's friend, but if you tend to suffer from cravings, it is an even more powerful tool. Research has shown that after as few as ten minutes of strenuous exercise the brain produces endorphins (the feel-good neurotransmitters) and serotonin which calm you down and decrease stress hormone levels. One of the best ways to silence a powerful craving is to go for a brisk walk, clear your head, and get the same sort of an injection of hormones you'd get from eating a sugary or fatty snack. Exercise also stimulates the evolutionary 'fight or flight' pathways in the brain that instantly switch off hunger messages (because in nature, there's no point worrying about food when you're running for your life). Even if you hate the thought of getting sweaty, stick at it. Exercise stimulates feel-good hormones so, over time, your brain will learn to see exercise as a reward.

For the Soother the essential first step is to carve out a ring-fenced period of time for exercise – book a regular class (pre-pay if possible to steel your resolve) and make sure it is an immovable item in your diary. Soothers are likely to be so busy looking after others that you will have become quite adept at making excuses for why you can't possibly do any exercise today. Add a tiny smattering of lethargy, fatigue or self-consciousness in to the mix and you've got an evening spent in front of the TV when you could and should be at the gym.

Soothers are probably not best advised to pick extreme sports or fiercely competitive forms of exercise. Instead look for more nurturing, gentle classes if you can (e.g. Pilates, stretch, meditation).

Not everyone is born sporty. Many of us associate exercise with embarrassment and discomfort. But you might be able to trick yourself into liking it by roping in a few friends and doing anything that gets you active together. And accept that the first ten minutes of any cardio exercise (the 'toxic ten') are horrid. However, it always gets easier after that, so grit your teeth and keep going.

Avoid the temptation to reward your exercise efforts with food: It is very tempting to end a tough session at the gym with a frothy coffee or an energy bar, but watch out! Studies show people typically overestimate calories burned relative to calories consumed, and you could be wiping out the benefits of all your efforts. Instead, make the most of your post-session shower and incorporate a different element of your beauty or grooming regime each time, so by the end of the week you'll feel fabulous and ready for the weekend.

Try wearing a pedometer or find your way around a good fitness calculating phone app, then aim is to achieve 10,000 steps a day, which roughly translates into walking 5 miles.

TRY BIKRAM YOGA

Studies have shown that yoga can reduce symptoms of depression, including focusing on negative feelings and the emotional eating. One study has found that Bikram yoga is powerfully effective in this regard, with devotees showing a threefold drop in stress and emotional eating after doing two classes a week for eight weeks (compared to non-yogis).[129]

Hot yoga is any class in a super-heated room, but traditional Bikram yoga is a set 90-minute class which takes you through 26 classical postures and two breathing exercises, all done in the same order in a 105 degree Celsius room. The postures are designed to stretch and strengthen the muscles, as well as compress and 'rinse' the organs of the body, and the heated room helps facilitate the release of toxins – you either love it or hate it. Fans say it leaves them feeling accomplished and totally high on endorphins afterwards. It is great for those who like structure and discipline – and while you're in there your head is completely clear and you can't possibly think of anything else.

Brief Soother summary

The Soother is a warm-hearted, reliable, generous and caring person but, through no fault of your own, you might have gradually developed an unhealthy relationship with food and a tendency to 'use' food to ease emotional discomfort, stress and boredom. The key to finding and maintaining a healthy weight lies in using more of your time and energy for *you*, and by setting a few simple boundaries and experimenting with the myriad other ways you can soothe yourself and others that don't require food and drink. Simple, easy steps like this will break the conditioned association of food and feeling good, in addition to diet plans that stabilise blood sugar levels.

If you do just one thing ...

Find other ways to feel warm and fuzzy inside and put yourself first – always. Because if you don't have good health and feel good about yourself you can't make the most of everything life has to offer. Ask yourself daily: 'What do I need to do to stay on track today?', and make that your first priority.

Chapter 13
The Traditional

Who is The Traditional?

Traditionals are dependable, reliable, stable and safe – perhaps a little too cautious at times – but you are friendly, popular and the absolute bedrock of your family or social circle.

You are the sort who loves to honour traditions, whether these are family, cultural or societal customs. You wouldn't miss your annual school mates' get-together for the world – it's a firm, non-negotiable diary entry. Christmas is also a favourite time of year, but all the commercialism irks you somewhat and you don't think it should just be about gifts – it's the time spent with family that's important. These celebrations and rituals offer a sense of grounded-ness which is important for your measure of belonging and security.

You're a stickler for following rules where possible – you'd drive around for ages rather than park illegally, complete your tax returns way before the deadline and have no issue with reprimanding other peoples' kids if they are far out of line. This is due to your strong sense of right and wrong and the apparent self-confidence that goes with it. This self-belief has many benefits, including being a good leader. This rigidity enables you to be decisive when you need to be – anyone would feel safe to have you as a captain of their ship.

But there are potential vulnerabilities here. Many Traditionals stick so rigidly to what they know as it feels safe and secure – new experiences bring about a rumble of apprehension which is frankly unenjoyable to a Traditional, rather than exciting as it would be for, say, a Rebel. You are very often utterly confounded by the ever-changing news reports – it can feel as if the goalposts just keep on moving. You much prefer to go to the same holiday resort every year, where you know proprietors of the local hotel. This is not because you are unadventurous – adventure definitely has its place and at times you can surprise others with your overt courage – but because the owners of the hotel are more like friends now and you'd feel guilty if you spent money elsewhere. You know how hard these people work to keep afloat. Traditionals know about tough times and quietly, surreptitiously find ways to help others.

You generally prefer life to be simple, straightforward and very much within set parameters. This doesn't mean you are unambitious, because your urge to follow instructions to the letter has meant you have moved efficiently up the ranks in your chosen career. From the outside, you seem cool as a cucumber and always in control. However, you're not brilliant with 'signals', so if someone thinks they can communicate with you by dropping hints, they're sorely mistaken.

You know what you like to eat and you think you know what's healthy and what's not. For the most part you stick with familiar foods and the meals you've always enjoyed, you really don't understand why you are gaining weight.

Classic Traditional eating behaviours

Routines and familiarity are important to the Traditional. You are likely to eat from a very small repertoire of set meals, with certain favourites on certain days. In limiting your dietary options you could be inadvertently putting yourself at risk of nutritional imbalance and too many fattening foods.

- **Childhood rules still apply.** Traditionals have a strong compulsion to stick to dietary rules established in childhood. You were probably brought up to eat whatever is put in front of you regardless of whether you like it, or whether you're full. This could develop into an unresponsive 'stop' mechanism, which means you eat more than your body really needs.
- **Snack attack.** You are likely to graze and snack between meals because you hate being 'hangry' and you believe you just can't function on an empty stomach because this is what you've been told your whole life. But the snacking calories are – for most of us – surplus to requirements. Worse, in providing a steady stream of sugar into your blood, you will be keeping your insulin levels topped up, and this means you could be putting your body in a permanent fat-storage mode.
- **Vegetable reluctance.** It is unlikely you manage the full five portions of fruit and vegetables a day, let alone the now recommended seven – partly because you might not have been introduced to a wide repertoire of options, or because you might have decided at an early age that you don't like certain vegetables, and that has been that.
- **Nursery food.** You like a carb-heavy existence which hikes your insulin levels, making cravings more likely and weight loss difficult.
- **Big breakfasts.** Most Traditionals couldn't contemplate starting the day without a big bowl of breakfast cereal and/or a couple of slices of toast with jam as this is what you've always done. Even if you're heeding the health warnings and you've switched from Cornflakes to Branflakes and white bread to brown, the classic British breakfast is so carbohydrate heavy it could be setting you up for a blood sugar spin and tough-to-resist cravings for the day.

Traditional case study

Stephen likes what he likes, and he knows exactly what this is.
He likes hearty food that fills him up, not things that he would be
embarrassed to pronounce. Stephens's wife has suggested he tries
to reduce the amount of carbohydrates he eats with every meal,
but he doesn't see why the meals that his mum made are suddenly
considered 'bad'. In fact, this 'advice' quite annoys Stephen. Even
though he knows Sarah is just trying to help, it feels like nagging.
And that doesn't get anyone anywhere!

Stephen knows he sounds like an old man when he moans
about how things keep changing. Sarah says he can't keep eating
the post-match-sized portions he did when he was in his 20s, as
he's now a 'midult' (what a ridiculous word that is anyway …).
It doesn't make sense to Stephen that he's doing what he's always
done and is now continually gaining weight. Yeah, maybe there
aren't as many kickabouts, and sure, the job is more office-based
than it used to be, but should that really matter so much? He eats
healthily – half the plate filled with starchy carbs, right? And who
doesn't have a pudding? That's simply part of the meal.

But … at the edges of his conscious mind Stephen knows he
can't carry on like this. His dad died of a heart attack in middle age
so there might be an inherited risk, but somehow this knowledge
makes the big changes that Sarah talks about even more terrifying.
Stephen only ever commits to things he knows he can do, and do
well; so what if he can't completely change himself with all these
new diet fads? The thought of change feels overwhelming, which
leaves Stephen finding even more solace in his well-trodden eating
and lifestyle patterns.

The Traditional's mind hacks

Shrinkology hacks for Traditionals are about gradually shifting your thinking outside the box. There are so many other shapes! Circles, triangles, ovals ... but you don't need to transform from a circle into a hexagon – rather, approach these hacks as gently nudging your parameters so that your circle becomes an oval. This will allow you to overcome ingrained habits and dietary myths so that you can arrive at a healthy weight for your body.

DAILY HACKS

Challenge your assumptions

Traditionals can have ingrained assumptions around food such as:

- 'This is what my mum cooked for me, so it must be the right thing to eat.'
- 'Eating fat can't be good, as fat is – well – fat!'
- 'It's rude not to clear your plate.'

Making assumptions can hold us back from seeing the full range of possibilities. It is very natural, but making them puts us at risk of failing to ask important questions – of ourselves, situations and others – because we think we already know the answers.

> If you're not careful, you can find that to assume = makes an 'ass' out of 'u' and 'me'.
>
> Making a point of noticing the assumptions you might be unconsciously making, and occasionally challenging them, is a great way to open your mind to potential new avenues of behaviour.

CHALLENGE YOUR BELIEFS

Each day, aim to pick one of your influential thoughts
to do with food and eating and ask yourself:
1. Where has this assumption stemmed from?
2. What's the logic behind this assumption?
3. What if the assumption wasn't true (or correct)?
4. What other things could occur if I chose to think
and act in a different way?
5. How can I prove/disprove this assumption,
i.e. what's the evidence for it?

If you take the example of 'dietary fat is bad', your answers
to the above questions might be:
1. 'It was always in the news – fat makes you fat.'
2. 'It makes total sense that when you eat fat it turns into
fat in your body.'
3. 'Perhaps eating fat is not the only reason why I'm
gaining weight.'
4. 'I love the taste of real butter, it would be fab to eat it
without feeling guilty.'
5. 'There were news stories about fat being bad for you,
but perhaps there's been more research that shows it's
not that simple. I could look into it more online and talk
to my GP.'

This exercise is not designed to criticise your assumptions but to make you aware that there might be alternative views, and perhaps healthier options – when it comes to diet and weight, they might just be helpful. It's good to break out of old habits sometimes.

As Henry Ford, the American founder of the Ford Motor Company once said: 'If you always do what you've always done, you'll always get what you've always got.'

Break out of the box with new rituals

Traditionals tend to love their habits and routines, and this isn't necessarily a bad thing – it puts you in a very strong position to utilise this sense of self-discipline to develop healthy new behavioural patterns.

Try playing with the idea of adopting one or two new rituals, just to see if you can release some of the associations that might be unwittingly tethering you to unhelpful old eating habits.

- Use brightly coloured cooking utensils to increase stimulation to create a novel food prep environment
- Sit at a different place at the table (see Eating on Autopilot on page 257)
- Use different plates (ideally smaller!)
- Play music, or unfamiliar music if you already listen to music when eating
- Try al-fresco dining (even if it means you have to wrap up warm).

Crisis control for cravings

Distraction equals subtraction

Although eating mindlessly means that some people scoff with little or no conscious knowledge, using distraction in an intentional way can curb food cravings. To appreciate how powerful distraction can be, think about how quickly time passes when you're on an intense session of Minecraft. If you're not into gaming, think about why using a handheld phone while driving is illegal – attending to the call, email or text distracts attention away from the road, which could be fatal. For Traditionals who need an immediate hack, you can halt your cravings with the following techniques:

- Organise a cupboard. If you're having a major craving crisis, take on an absorbing task such as spring-cleaning your wardrobe. This will occupy all of your attention as you decide what possessions to keep, discard or store away. As a Traditional you're practical in nature so this hack will feel satisfying and purposeful.
- Do some DIY. This takes planning, research and patience, all of which can act as useful distractions.
- Call on your inner devil. If your house is practically perfect already (which wouldn't be unusual for a Traditional), think about one of your best friends. Now, devise a clever prank that you can play on him or her. Consider where you would do it, how it could be set up, what you'd need to do to maintain the joke until its punchline. Just make sure it's not a cream pie type prank as that could negate all your hard distraction work.
- Think about the best kiss you could ever have. No more needs to be said here …

While you're distracting yourself, the amount of food you would have consumed is subtracted from your day. The key here is to distract yourself purposefully and intentionally so that your attention is consumed with the task.

When you're alone

Make a bucket list

Even though the Traditional loves order and routine, there will very often still be a part of you that will be daydreaming about more. To start to nurture your adventurous side, simply sit down and ask yourself: 'What might it feel like if I ...?'

- ... went to these places. These can be far afield like countries on the opposite side of the planet or places closer to home. Perhaps both!
- ... tried these hobbies. List activities you've always had a secret curiosity about, which can be active such as horse riding or activities you can do at home such as big wool knitting.
- ... embarked on new experiences. There are loads of companies that specialise in 'experiences' such as racing a Formula One car, sky diving (yes, you could do it!) and hot air ballooning. New experiences at home could be watching a genre of movie you wouldn't have previously chosen, playing different board games with family or even trying adult LEGO®.

Even if you don't try all of the things on your list, simply thinking about them and writing them down is a good way to let your mind and imagination flow. Having your dreams and aspirations written down explicitly can help you meet your goals, particularly when they are closely aligned.

Quick fix

Stop at the red lights

Studies show the power of the colour red to signal 'stop' goes well beyond the roads, as people eat and drink less from red glasses and plates.[130] As a Traditional, you have a soft spot for rules and laws, so playing with colour can be a fun and easy fix to integrate in your everyday meals.

- Find red plates – your brain unconsciously is thinking about stopping, which in turn will reduce the amount you eat.
- Change light bulbs wherever you happen to eat from clear to blue. A study by a group of researchers from the Food Scientists Department of the University of Arkansas found that blue lighting made food appear less pleasant compared eating in a white or yellow lit room. This perception resulted in men consuming less food, although women didn't appear affected.[131] If you're a male Traditional, go down to the DIY shop and invest in some blue lights.
- Use a dimmer switch to lower the lighting in a room can also relax the mind and body.

Do your homework
(slow-build, longer-term hacks)

Nudge your boundaries with SMART goals

In the quest for change – if you are prepared to see that change is useful here – it is important that the Traditional takes things really slowly, one baby step at a time. The key is to make a SMART plan – and there's nothing more the Traditional loves than a plan!

If your aim is steady weight loss and being able to stay at a healthy weight without undue effort or hunger, it helps to establish your goals and make sure they are SMART.

- Specific – vague goals such as 'I want to be slimmer/fitter/healthier' are difficult to pin down as they are subjective and mean different things to different people. A goal of losing a stone in weight is much more specific.
- Measurable – a specific goal is much easier to measure as you work your way in the right direction, so you can keep your motivation high by monitoring each pound as it falls away.
- Achievable – a smart goal should be realistic for you and your circumstances as unmet goals can suck the motivation out of even the most determined Traditional. Instead of picking one big goal ('I will get back into my jeans') choose smaller, bite-sized and achievable goals ('I will drop one jeans size in the next month'), which will help boost motivation and confidence. Once some small goals are met, bigger ones can be set.
- Relevant – ask yourself if the goal you have picked really is relevant to you. Do you really want to be able to wear something that you've never worn before? What's a true healthy weight for you (see page 89)? Trying to make health changes to please others or in order to fit in with some false concept of who you want to be could make changes difficult to maintain long term.

- Timely – is this a good time to embark on a behavioural change? If so, give yourself a realistic timeframe. A healthy weight loss is around one to two pounds per week, so it might take three and a half months to lose a stone. This goal might be more 'achievable' if it's broken down into mini goals (such as 'I will lose four pounds in a month') – and make sure you give yourself huge pat on the back when you get there.

Before you start on a SMART weight-loss or weight-maintenance plan, ask yourself a few questions:

- WHAT SITUATIONS/CONTEXTS/TIMES MIGHT TIP ME BACK INTO OLD HABITS? Home? Work? Being with parents? When I finish work for the day? Look back at your food/mood diary for answers.
- WHAT CAN I ACHIEVE IN TERMS OF MAKING HEALTHIER FOOD CHOICES? Can I reduce portions; eat more veg; limit second helpings?
- WHAT COULD MAKE TRYING NEW FOODS EASIER FOR ME? The support of my spouse; taking a walk at lunchtime; using different cutlery and crockery

Now think about setting small, specific goals which will take you in the right direction and ultimately lead to your overall goal. What about aiming simply to integrate new foods and experiences into your healthy eating goals? This is a great one for the Traditional as it will help ease you out of safe, familiar habits and encourage you to consider developing new patterns. See the Shrinkology Science section on page 126 to find out how to become a healthy 'doer', whether that's a regular vegetable eater or a regular exerciser.

TRY THIS SMALL, SPECIFIC, SMART GOAL:

- **S**pecific goal – I will try one new fruit and one new vegetable a week.
- **M**easurable – this is easy to record in your food diary (see Chapter 5). Also jot down how it feels to try these new foods – are you surprised by the tastes? How does trying this make you feel? Note all this new information in your food/mood diary.
- **A**chievable – this goal should be achievable but you may need to do a little research about different kinds of produce – involve your family here as it can be exciting to try new things together. There may be markets or farms nearby that you can explore.
- **R**elevant – remind yourself why you want to maintain a healthy weight, i.e. why is it important to you?
- **T**imely – when trying something new like this, it's good to check in with the goal at the end of the first week. Do you want to keep going? Step up this goal (two of each?) or set a new goal?
  Don't forget to give yourself a pat on the back for achieving the goal you set!

At the end of the week look back at your diary and compare it to your initial food/mood journal. You may well find that how you feel about eating is starting to change already.

Eating on Autopilot

We all have limited 'cognitive capacity'. In other words, our brains are much like computers in the sense that processing capability and memory storage are finite. This may seem extraordinary considering the complexity of tasks we achieve every single day. Take driving, for instance – we simultaneously have to observe the environment around us that's constantly and quickly changing, respond to these changes in a split second and still keep in mind where we're going and which direction to take.

Complex tasks like this are made possible by the fact that certain repetitive behaviours become automatic. Once we learn to drive, we don't explicitly think about pushing our foot down on the brake when we see a car slow in front of us – we do it without conscious thought processes. Automatic processes come about when we carry out a behaviour on a regular basis, so it's not surprising that something we do every day of our lives – such as eating – is swiftly set to autopilot so the brain can be occupied doing other things to save valuable cognitive resources.

This autopilot mode explains how habits are formed. A set habit will emerge in contexts that have stability and familiarity (such as the home) and it will evolve from actions that take place frequently (such as eating or drinking). It doesn't take much repetition, and before long you might find your little ways of choosing and consuming food have become deeply ingrained.

For instance, if we pull a pizza out of the freezer and pop it in the oven we can do so on autopilot while of thinking about work or family or something completely different.

Context is an important factor, and this is why we can find ourselves stuck in a familiar, repetitive breakfast rut. In general, we eat our first meal of the day at home. The Traditional is probably more likely than other Shrinkology types to eat lunch and dinner at home too because you prefer your habitual and favourite meals.

But this factor alone is one reason why Traditionals might find unhelpful eating habits harder to break.

The Traditional might eat lunch somewhere easy, such as a work-based canteen, or you might take a sandwich to the office – think about it: you probably choose from a very narrow range of options. And as we explained early in this chapter, those habitual choices might be unwittingly holding you back from finding or maintaining a healthy weight.

So, think about your SMART goals and consider stretching outside your comfort zone to try new foods and meals, and perhaps set up more helpful new habits. The key for Traditionals is that this process should happen in a controlled way that feels manageable, which can include shaking up not only what you eat but also the eating context itself (see page 254).

Because we know how important context is to our behaviour, making changes in your environment can really help to break the habits of a lifetime.

Traditional's eat-less tips and tricks

Traditionals, by definition, tend to be creatures of habit. An obedient adherence to rules and convention means you'll eat when you get up in the morning, in the middle of the day and again in the evening, regardless of what you might have nibbled, snacked and grazed in-between, and regardless of whether you're hungry or not. But after years of habitual eating like this you could have lost sight of just how much food your body really needs.

To you, breakfast is a non-negotiable. You will always tuck into a bowl of cereal or a couple of slices of toast automatically, without thinking, as part of set pattern of an ordinary day. You have a cereal favourite and at weekends you might throw in a couple of slices of (white) toast spread with Flora and marmalade. You might treat yourself to a couple of biscuits with morning coffee (which is always at 11am and never sooner or later) that could even be black coffee ('healthier'). Then a sandwich for lunch, and the evening meal will be one of very few options then a mini meal of toast or cereal before bed. Traditionals should pay close attention to the Shrinkology Fundamentals in Chapter 6, as there is much you can learn! You are very likely still eating the large portion sizes you enjoyed in your teens/twenties, when your calorie needs are now dropping, so take note of the plate sizes/portion control hints and tips.

- Polish up your satiety signalling. **Learn to listen to fullness triggers more carefully. It is so important to learn what proper hungry actually feels like and to understand that you can push through it and get quite happily through to the other side without a full sit-down meal or substantial snack.**
- Your food diary is crucial. **Check the hunger scales on page 60 and ask yourself, are you really hungry every time you eat? Just how full are you when you finish eating?**
- Expand your vegetable horizons. **You might be a meat and two veg character, but the rules have changed and you're going to have to up your vegetable game. As we explained in Chapter 6 a wide variety of different vegetables each day provides you with a super-healthy spread of plant nutrients, and is the healthiest possible way to fill you up and help you achieve your happy, healthy weight. To achieve this goal most Traditionals will have to push outside that established comfort zone – instead of apples, grapes and tangerines, cabbage and carrots, aim to try a different, unfamiliar vegetable or fruit every week.**
- Revisit the vegetables you thought you hated as a child **(broad beans, cabbage?). Experiment with new ways to prepare and cook them – you'll be surprised how your old vegetable nemeses collection can be transformed by olive oil and a sprinkling of spices.**

- Consider going 'slightly' vegetarian. Ease yourself in to reducing your dietary reliance on meat gradually by instigating 'meat-free Mondays' or one vegetarian day (any day) each week.
- Become a vegetable ninja. Take a tip from parenting guides for veg-refusenik toddlers and grate courgette, carrots, cauliflower or broccoli into sauces, casseroles, salads and even sandwiches. You won't notice but you'll have upped your veg and nutrition count immeasurably.

VEGETABLE MAKEOVER

- Stir-fry cabbage with oil, salt and sesame seeds
- Roast cauliflower florets with turmeric, salt and pepper
- Halve Brussels sprouts and fry with pancetta, or grate into a tangily dressed salad
- Mash sweet potato or celeriac instead of white potatoes
- Mash a tin of black beans into meatballs or burgers
- Serve buttery mashed butter beans as you would mash
- Make cauliflower 'rice' (grate or blend raw) and courgette spaghetti
- Try seductive salads: There's so much more to salad than lettuce, tomatoes and cucumber and it's not just a summer side dish; winter salads are really good too. They are a really good way for the Traditional to go crazy in the salad aisle and get adventurous with salad bowls, exotic slaws and wilted warm salads. Ease yourself into a host of potentially bitter new flavours with tangy homemade salad dressings packed with healthy oils and spices.

- Try vegetable anchoring. Link an item of fruit or vegetables to a set behaviour you already do every day to 'anchor' it and create a healthful new habit. Grab an apple on the school run each morning, or order a salad with your lunchtime sandwich.
- Aim to change your approach to sugar. Make familiar puddings and sweets an occasional indulgence rather than the compulsory end to a meal. Make life easier by weaning yourself off gradually, switching to fruit-based desserts, or substituting dessert for a piece of cheese with an apple. Then work towards making pudding a once-a-week treat with your big Sunday roast, and enjoy it without restriction. Some Traditions are very definitely worth keeping!
- Aim to reduce your reliance on takeaways and ready meals. The Traditional might rather enjoy the 'we always have a takeaway on a Friday', or the 'it's kebabs after the pub quiz' convention. But even supposedly healthy ready meals aren't really healthy and, with practice and a little clever shopping, you can rustle up a nutritious home-cooked meal in the time it takes to warm up a packet meal in the microwave. And if you batch-cook and fill your freezer, you can create delicious ready meals of your own.
- Investigate cookery courses. At the very least, find a cookbook with slightly out-of-your-comfort zone recipes which inspire you. Following TV recipe programmes might broaden your culinary horizons and help 'normalise' unconventional, or what you might consider to be slightly exotic, food choices.
- No more diet foods. In a long-standing concession to weight loss you may well have acquired a cupboard full of 'diet' foods – slimline tonic, 'light' margarine, 0% fat yoghurts, and there could be diet-ready meals in tins or in the freezer. This might be well-meaning, but it doesn't fit the Shrinkology plan. Studies show chemically processed 'frankenfoods' (even ones with 'diet' labelling) could actually be making it harder for you to lose weight (see Chapter 2).

Your body will be much better able to fine-tune hunger signalling when it isn't being bamboozled by artificial colourings, flavourings, thickeners and sweeteners.

- Try switching to plain (natural) full-fat Greek yoghurt. Make the switch from 0% fat 'fruit' yoghurt and measure the difference in time before you feel hungry again. Studies show the fat content fills us up more quickly and keeps us feeling fuller for longer, leading to a healthier weight long term. Natural yoghurt has an intense natural sweetness that really doesn't need sugar, honey or sweeteners which are absolutely essential to disguise the thin, sour tang of diet yoghurts. Also it's delicious.

- Aim to break the white bread habit. Some Traditionals will still be steadfastly hanging onto the white sliced bread of their childhood. Surely the fibre message is getting through now? No one questions the fact that high-fibre carbohydrates which release energy slowly – brown rice, pasta and bread – will slow the insulin response that puts you at risk of type 2 diabetes. Whole grains also boost your fibre intake, delivering nutrients, food for your gut bacteria, and a faster 'throughput' which helps protect you from bowel cancer. If you or your Traditional household insists on everything white, try going part wholegrain with the 50/50 options available in bread, bagels, wraps, pasta, noodles and crackers. The taste is very similar, and from here, a shift to full wholegrain will be a small step away.

TRADITIONAL SOCIAL MEDIA SOS

If you're a great fan of social media you'll know that checking Facebook, Instagram and Twitter can be really bad for self-image and ultimately for weight management. The best route for the Traditional – because you're a sucker for rigid rules – is to try setting a few self-imposed social media limits. Create house rules or a contract to be negotiated equally and agreed so everyone is happy.

Try 'no phones' when talking to anyone, never at the table, never before saying good morning to your partner, never on a walk … And aim to create technology havens in your home where screens have to be turned off (bedrooms, bathrooms, or the family dinner table).

The Traditional's diet digest

The Traditional's love of convention and mistrust of the new means you are unlikely to dip your toe in the water of the fad diets which crop up each year. You just don't have the conviction to believe that a green juice provides you with a better breakfast than toast.

Many Traditionals might struggle with intermittent fasting because you hate to be hungry and you find it super-hard to shake off. Don't beat yourself up if the raw food diets, 'clean eating', cabbage soup or lemon juice diets didn't work, and if you just can't bring yourself to join the ranks of Paleo aficionados who start their day with offal or steak.

You might find yourself intrigued by the science behind the Mediterranean diet – numerous different studies have shown that consumption of fresh fish, vegetables, salads, fruit, olive oil and nuts (as well as red wine) have significantly beneficial effects on heart health and can aid weight loss. But the broad advice to embrace Mediterranean foods probably works best for Shrinkology types who detest the confines of calorie counting and structured meal plans (such as a Gourmet). Most Traditionals feel more comfortable when working with a clearly defined set of dietary rules they can trust and believe in. It would be all too easy for the Traditional to descend into a Mediterranean twilight world where salted peanuts tick the nuts box (they don't), baked beans count as pulses (the sauce is packed with sugar, so it's not the best option) and fish fingers supply all your omega-3 fatty acids (you really need to be eating a portion or two of oily fish such as salmon or mackerel each week).

As a Traditional you are most likely to find your best chance of success with a diet that is backed by solid, robust, believable science, and which is clearly structured. As a first port of call, check out the NHS Choices website (www.nhs.co.uk) which has clear, simple dietary advice written by qualified dietitians. You'll find additional advice about cutting back on sugar, and about generally eating less to create that all important calorie deficit.

However, it is worth noting that any public health advice like this has to be created to appeal to a mass audience so it is based on long-established principles and made super-simple for everyone to understand. In the last twenty years there have been huge advances in nutritional research with study after study questioning the appropriateness of the Government's 'Eatwell Plate'. So it is important to keep an open mind if you can – your personalised hacks will help!

You might find success by joining a local Weight Watchers or Slimming World group. They are similar in that you pay a nominal amount to attend each week, and in return you receive advice and guidance on healthy eating, and your weight is recorded. Their methods are different. Weight Watchers works by allocating 'points' to an item of food or a meal and urging you to keep within a set points total each day. The advantage is you can eat EVERYTHING, no food is banned, but you just have to do the maths. If you choose to use up all your points on a portion of sticky toffee pudding, you'll end up hungrily chewing celery or undressed salad later. You don't even have to keep track of your points as there's an app to do it for you. You'll also be allocated more points if you regularly exercise.

Slimming World works by dividing foods into two categories: 'free foods' (such as plain pasta or vegetables) which you can eat, er, freely, and 'syns' (sauces, fats, treats) which you should limit in your quest to lose weight.

Both methods can really help if you have quite a bit of weight to lose – their numerous happy weight loss stories are testament to their success. But it is important to be aware that their success depends, partly, on our human failings and the fact that the vast majority of slimming club slimmers will regain their lost weight. If you choose this route to weight loss don't be so blinded by your success that you fail to absorb the importance of the long-term plan. Maintaining your happy healthy weight, when you get there, will require a fresh look at Shrinkology Fundamentals and a certain degree of self-discipline to keep you eating healthily, even without the incentive of a weekly weigh-in.

Traditional tips to cut back on the booze

A classic Traditional drinking scenario: the favourite pint at the favourite chair at the favourite pub **or** the great big glass of red wine sitting in your favourite chair in front of the TV every evening. You can take one big step towards better managing your weight if you can grasp control of your habitual drinking. Try these targeted tips:

• Once unhelpful bad habits are formed, the brain stops thinking about it, leaving you with routines that are performed on autopilot, below your conscious radar. Shake up your drinking routine. Change the chairs around in your living room so yours is no longer next to a side table, or nip to the gym in the evening to minimise TV drinking time (and make it much less likely you'll round off the evening with alcohol).

• Pour your soft drink of choice into your favourite crystal wine glass and enjoy all the positives of the tactile associations, the sense of reward – without the booze.

• As a Traditional you're more likely to be a 'stopper' than a 'starter'. So, the best way to curtail your drinking is to decide ahead of time how many drinks you are planning to have, making the decision to stop when you've reached your self-imposed limit.

• Traditionals love a bit of logic and reason, so when a booze craving strikes try a little no drinking mathematics. If a glass of wine or a pint of beer costs around £5 you are saving more than £30 for every week you abstain. Keep that up for a month and you not only reap the benefits of weight loss, great skin, clearer eyes and better sleep but you'll be considerably wealthier.

• If you do manage to cut down on drinking, or even go completely alcohol-free for a while, do remember to reinforce your abstinence success by celebrating it.

The Traditional's tailored exercise prescription

Exercise for the Traditional doesn't have to be a burden. It can be simple, even enjoyable – and you don't need to do much to make an impact. Your love of predictability and routine means you might enjoy physical activities where there is an emphasis on mind-body connection, those that involve little risk and are inherently self-focused.

The key to creating a successful personalised exercise plan lies in applying SMART goals (see page 254). Ensure your exercise plan is manageable (start at a pace and time that are slightly more than what you think you can do, then increase by small increments each week); convenient (make it as easy as possible to be active throughout the day); repeatable (it should be easy, efficient and, ideally, enjoyable); incremental (you are more likely to stick at an activity when you get a sense of progress); and measureable. You should be able to measure how much exercise you've done, and your progress should be visible at all times. Use a workbook or an app on your smartphone. If swimming takes your fancy, set yourself the aim to swim a mile (or a half marathon) in laps, ticking them off one by one.

Many Traditionals favour solo activities like running and cycling. These are not just types of exercise, they are also an incredibly cheap and efficient means of transport. Try drawing a 1-mile circle around your house and creating a self-imposed rule that you will always walk if you're going anywhere within that circle. Now draw a 5-mile circle for cycling. If your chosen form of exercise gets you from A to B efficiently and cost-effectively, the raised heart rate and pumping muscles are just a bonus.

Slip into exercise gear *before* you shower when you wake up in the morning. Studies show if your willpower is weak, you're more likely to get to the gym or jump on the exercise bike if you can tick it off your list before you get distracted by anything else. It means you

TRY IYENGAR YOGA

There's a form of yoga to suit every Shrinkology type, and for Traditionals an excellent yoga entry point would be Iyengar (sometimes also called 'Hatha'). This is a slow and thoughtful class and a great form of yoga for anyone who might be put off by the more spiritual elements they might have heard about. It's also a great way to learn breathing techniques that can help in times of stress.

This form of yoga puts emphasis on getting into postures with correct alignment and holding them rather than flowing through different poses. It is often a gentle yoga class which uses set postures to restore balance and flexibility to the body while utilising a variety of props (belts, blocks and pillow-like bolsters) to help beginners get into poses with correct alignment, even when they're new, injured or simply stiff. Sometimes there are even short Savasanas (time of rest) between each pose to ensure you reap the full benefits.

It lacks the dance-like, free-flowing qualities of other kinds of yoga posses and some people might find it a little too slow, but it's a great starting point for anyone new to yoga.

are primed and ready for activity (if you're wearing trainers you're more likely to walk fast or even jog, and take the stairs rather than the escalator) and other people's comments ('have you been for a run?') will serve as a constant reminder to get on with it.

Book a physical challenge: find a Park Run (these are timed, friendly 5k free events that take place in local parks on Saturdays at 9am all over the world – you can walk, jog, run, bring the dogs or a baby in the pram (see www.parkrun.com). Or try a 5k Tough Mudder race (see www.nuclear-races.co.uk), a bike ride, or even a half marathon – the key is to set your sights on something that pushes you beyond your current capabilities and out of your comfort zone.

Traditionals love exercise which has a practical element or which allows them to kill two birds with one stone. Gardening is a great example – a fantastically calorie-burning strength-builder which also (bonus!) ensures your garden looks fantastic.

Brief Traditional summary

Traditionals are they type of person everyone wants around – you're a 'rock'. But if your weight is bothering you, it might be time to shake things up a bit and explore new eating patterns and activities. Don't think of broadening your horizons as being disloyal to the past – it's simply an exciting way to ensure you are making your future as healthy and varied as possible.

If you do just one thing ...

Muster up your inner curiosity and try new things – experiment with one new and unfamiliar piece of fruit and vegetable every week. You might be surprised by what you can learn to like!

Part Four
Shrinkology for Life

Now you know your Shrinkology type you are all
set to create your very own personalized Shrinkology
Solution. But one factor that sets Shrinkology apart
from other weight-loss approaches is its flexibility,
which means it can be for life. Circumstances
change, we all get older, life throws up curveballs,
and Shrinkology is cleverly designed to adapt so
that the principles – and support – stay with you
whatever happens now and into the future.

Chapter 14
Your Shrinkology Future

If you're reading this chapter, you've probably diligently read through most of this book rather than surreptitiously swiping tips from your Shrinkology type. Hooray! We confidently believe you will have already found Shrinkology thinking useful, and although there is no super-quick diet fix, we hope you go on to discover that a Shrinktastic mindset is incredibly empowering and the best way to ensure you find and maintain a healthy weight.

We also recommend you dip in and out of this book in the future, because all the evidence suggests that your Shrinkology type will change over time. Your circumstances, responsibilities and perceptions can alter dramatically throughout the course of your life as you are influenced by changing circumstance and the complexities of the ageing process.

Psychologists and researchers used to think that our personality was formed in childhood and pretty much set, but recent research is challenging this long-held view. It seems that important traits like self-confidence, perseverance, conscientiousness, originality and the desire to excel can change[132] – for better or for worse, and this can have an impact on your Shrinkology type. Studies show different aspects of personality appear to develop through childhood, teens and early adulthood, stabilising at midlife, before gradually shifting again when we reach older adulthood. This makes sense when we consider personality in terms of our roles and responsibilities, which are generally more demanding in midlife when we frequently have to juggle family, career and whatever else.

The only trait that seems more likely to remain consistent throughout life is the stability of your moods (how likely you are to fly off the handle at any given provocation).

This means that although you might believe you were born a Rebel or your family life channelled you squarely down the Traditional route, you can quite easily find that a new job, the buzz of a demanding career, or pregnancy and the influx of young children may transform you into a Scrambler overnight. You also might find years of dieting have highlighted Magpie traits as you dip in and out of the latest diet ideologies, but through the influence of Shrinkology you could start to adopt more stable and helpful Traditional habits.

For any Shrinkology type, a protracted period of illness might nudge you closer to the Traditional dietary values of your childhood, or an unforeseen trauma (bereavement or divorce, perhaps) could bring out previously hidden Rebel tendencies. Equally, women might find the menopause heralds more of a Soother state of mind.

That's why we urge you to periodically return to Shrinkology, re-take the quiz, ask loved ones to answer the questions on your behalf, to see if you fit more comfortably into a different category now. This way you can keep up with the best diet plans to suit your evolving needs and try out new tips and hacks to support these changes.

The plasticity which allows our personality traits to naturally alter and shift throughout life also means we can purposefully change – if we want to. Studies show even a short, two-week course of therapy is enough to bring about long-term changes for the better.[133]

Simply knowing your personality is open to change can help reduce levels of anxiety and depression and improve your sense of behaviour control.[134]

You really can choose whether you want to hold on tight to your perfectionist Magpie traits or your hot-headed Rebel reactions or whether you'd prefer to cherry pick a few aspects of another Shrinkology type you admire or find potentially useful.

We all have the ability to see the world through different eyes, endure difficulties and take new paths. Even a tricky past, present and future experiences can be navigated with this new set of tools – and there's nothing to stop you from adding more and more Shrinkology hacks to your repertoire. That's the beauty of this flexible plan – you can build it exactly as you please.

There are thousands of different diets already out there, and novel, original and sometimes bonkers new regimes appearing all the time. Your solid foundation in Shrinkology should equip you to sift through and filter out the ones least likely to work for you, and pick up on potentially helpful elements that might. Knowing which ones are more likely to offer long-term healthy and stable eating behaviours and the right weight *for you*, can take much of the frustration out of dieting. Even if you crave short-term results, by keeping your eye on the long-term objective and using eating plans that suit *you*, you can break the cycle of dieting. Remember to keep using the website: www.shrinkology.co.uk and our social media feeds for verdicts on the latest diets, and whether they suit your type.

If you've started to experiment with the array of hacks described in your type chapter, you may have already realised that Shrinkology can benefit much more than your eating behaviour and weight. Many of the hacks will help you manage stress more effectively, take a more mindful approach to life and develop a sense of self-acceptance. This will enable you ensure your life becomes a little more grounded and calm and it should help you stay focused on the positives, as well as cope better with any negatives that will inevitably appear.

Shrinkology could be the key to finding and sticking at your happy, healthy weight long term. It could also be your first step in a sustained course of personal development that could significantly benefit your personal, social and even your working life long into the future.

Endnotes

1 Sacks, F.M., Bray, G.A., Carey, V.J., Smith, S.R., Ryan, D.H., Anton, S.D., McManus, K., Champagne, C.M., Bishop, L.M., Laranjo, N. and Leboff, M.S., 2009. Comparison of weight-loss diets with different compositions of fat, protein, and carbohydrates. *New England Journal of Medicine, 360*(9), pp.859–873.

2 http://digital.nhs.uk/catalogue/PUB23742

3 Scaglioni, S., Salvioni, M. and Galimberti, C., 2008. Influence of parental attitudes in the development of children eating behaviour. *British Journal of Nutrition, 99*(S1), pp.S22–S25.

4 Kelder, S.H., Perry, C.L., Klepp, K.I. and Lytle, L.L., 1994. Longitudinal tracking of adolescent smoking, physical activity, and food choice behaviors. *American journal of public health, 84*(7), pp.1121–1126.

5 Nicklas, T.A., 1995. Dietary studies of children and young adults (1973–1988): the Bogalusa Heart Study. *The American journal of the medical sciences, 310*, pp.S101–S108.

6 Birch, L.L. and Marlin, D.W., 1982. I don't like it; I never tried it: effects of exposure on two-year-old children's food preferences. *Appetite, 3*(4), pp.353–360.

7 Wardle, J., Herrera, M.L., Cooke, L. and Gibson, E.L., 2003. Modifying children's food preferences: the effects of exposure and reward on acceptance of an unfamiliar vegetable. *European journal of clinical nutrition, 57*(2), pp.341–348.

8 Francis, J.A., Stewart, S.H. and Hounsell, S., 1997. Dietary restraint and the selective processing of forbidden and nonforbidden food words. *Cognitive Therapy and Research, 21*(6), pp.633–646.

9 Polivy, J., Coleman, J. and Herman, C.P., 2005. The effect of deprivation on food cravings and eating behavior in restrained and unrestrained eaters. *International Journal of Eating Disorders, 38*(4), pp.301–309.

10 Herman, C.P. and Mack, D., 1975. Restrained and unrestrained eating. *Journal of personality, 43*(4), pp.647–660.

11 Lustig, R.H., Sen, S., Soberman, J.E. and Velasquez-Mieyer, P.A., 2004. Obesity, leptin resistance, and the effects of insulin reduction. *International journal of obesity, 28*(10), pp.1344–1348.

12 Lustig, R.H., 2006. Childhood obesity: behavioral aberration or biochemical drive? Reinterpreting the First Law of Thermodynamics. *Nature Reviews Endocrinology, 2*(8), pp.447–458.

13 Kalliomäki, M., Collado, M.C., Salminen, S. and Isolauri, E., 2008. Early differences in fecal microbiota composition in children may predict overweight. *The American journal of clinical nutrition, 87*(3), pp.534–538.

14 Maslowski, K.M. and Mackay, C.R., 2011. Diet, gut microbiota and immune responses. *Nature immunology, 12*(1), pp.5–9.

15 Suez, J., Korem, T., Zeevi, D., Zilberman-Schapira, G., Thaiss, C.A., Maza, O., Israeli, D., Zmora, N., Gilad, S., Weinberger, A. and Kuperman, Y., 2014. Artificial sweeteners induce glucose intolerance by altering the gut microbiota. Nature, 514(7521), pp.181–186.

16 Mäkivuokko, H., Tiihonen, K., Tynkkynen, S., Paulin, L. and Rautonen, N., 2010. The effect of age and non-steroidal anti-inflammatory drugs on human intestinal microbiota composition. British journal of nutrition, 103(02), pp.227–234.

17 Dethlefsen, L., Huse, S., Sogin, M.L. and Relman, D.A., 2008. The pervasive effects of an antibiotic on the human gut microbiota, as revealed by deep 16S rRNA sequencing. PLoS biol, 6(11), p.e280.

18 Compare, D., Coccoli, P., Rocco, A., Nardone, O.M., De Maria, S., Cartenì, M. and Nardone, G., 2012. Gut–liver axis: the impact of gut microbiota on non alcoholic fatty liver disease. Nutrition, Metabolism and Cardiovascular Diseases, 22(6), pp.471–476.

19 Cryan, J.F. and Dinan, T.G., 2012. Mind-altering microorganisms: the impact of the gut microbiota on brain and behaviour. Nature reviews neuroscience, 13(10), pp.701–712.

20 Galley, J.D. and Bailey, M.T., 2014. Impact of stressor exposure on the interplay between commensal microbiota and host inflammation. Gut Microbes, 5(3), pp.390–396.

21 Sidenvall, B., Nydahl, M. and Fjellström, C., 2000. The meal as a gift—the meaning of cooking among retired women. Journal of applied gerontology, 19(4), pp.405–423.

22 Cota, D., Tschöp, M.H., Horvath, T.L. and Levine, A.S., 2006. Cannabinoids, opioids and eating behavior: the molecular face of hedonism?. Brain research reviews, 51(1), pp.85–107.

23 K Garber, A. and H Lustig, R., 2011. Is fast food addictive?. Current drug abuse reviews, 4(3), pp.146–162.

24 Newman, J. and Taylor, A., 1992. Effect of a means-end contingency on young children's food preferences. Journal of experimental child psychology, 53(2), pp.200–216.

25 Just, D.R. and Price, J., 2013. Using incentives to encourage healthy eating in children. Journal of Human resources, 48(4), pp.855–872.

26 Kessler, H.S., 2016. Simple interventions to improve healthy eating behaviors in the school cafeteria. Nutrition reviews, 74(3), pp.198–209.

27 Cash, T.F., Thériault, J. and Annis, N.M., 2004. Body image in an interpersonal context: Adult attachment, fear of intimacy and social anxiety. Journal of social and clinical psychology, 23(1), pp.89–103.

28 Mandel, N. and Smeesters, D., 2008. The sweet escape: Effects of mortality salience on consumption quantities for high-and low-self-esteem consumers. Journal of Consumer Research, 35(2), pp.309–323.

29 Cheng, H.L. and Mallinckrodt, B., 2009. Parental bonds, anxious attachment, media internalization, and body image dissatisfaction: Exploring a mediation model. *Journal of Counseling Psychology*, 56(3), p.365.

30 Adam, T.C. and Epel, E.S., 2007. Stress, eating and the reward system. *Physiology & behavior*, 91(4), pp.449–458.

31 De Schipper, J.C., Oosterman, M. and Schuengel, C., 2012. Temperament, disordered attachment, and parental sensitivity in foster care: differential findings on attachment security for shy children. *Attachment & human development*, 14(4), pp.349–365.

32 Evers, C., Marijn Stok, F. and de Ridder, D.T., 2010. Feeding your feelings: Emotion regulation strategies and emotional eating. *Personality and Social Psychology Bulletin*, 36(6), pp.792–804.

33 Martyn-Nemeth, P., Penckofer, S., Gulanick, M., Velsor-Friedrich, B. and Bryant, F.B., 2009. The relationships among self-esteem, stress, coping, eating behavior, and depressive mood in adolescents. *Research in nursing & health*, 32(1), pp.96–109.

34 Ghosh, S., Laxmi, T.R. and Chattarji, S., 2013. Functional connectivity from the amygdala to the hippocampus grows stronger after stress. *Journal of Neuroscience*, 33(17), pp.7234–7244.

35 Gupta, R., Koscik, T.R., Bechara, A. and Tranel, D., 2011. The amygdala and decision-making. *Neuropsychologia*, 49(4), pp.760–766.

36 Youssef, F.F., Dookeeram, K., Basdeo, V., Francis, E., Doman, M., Mamed, D., Maloo, S., Degannes, J., Dobo, L., Ditshotlo, P. and Legall, G., 2012. Stress alters personal moral decision making. *Psychoneuroendocrinology*, 37(4), pp.491–498.

37 Starcke, K., Polzer, C., Wolf, O.T. and Brand, M., 2011. Does stress alter everyday moral decision-making?. *Psychoneuroendocrinology*, 36(2), pp.210–219.

38 Wansink, B. and Sobal, J., 2007. Mindless eating: the 200 daily food decisions we overlook. *Environment and Behavior*, 39(1), pp.106–123.

39 Koball, A.M., Meers, M.R., Storfer-Isser, A., Domoff, S.E. and Musher-Eizenman, D.R., 2012. Eating when bored: revision of the emotional eating scale with a focus on boredom. *Health psychology*, 31(4), p.521.

40 Guyenet, S.J. and Schwartz, M.W., 2012. Regulation of food intake, energy balance, and body fat mass: implications for the pathogenesis and treatment of obesity. *The Journal of Clinical Endocrinology & Metabolism*, 97(3), pp.745–755.

41 Hatori, M., Vollmers, C., Zarrinpar, A., DiTacchio, L., Bushong, E.A., Gill, S., Leblanc, M., Chaix, A., Joens, M., Fitzpatrick, J.A. and Ellisman, M.H., 2012. Time-restricted feeding without reducing caloric intake prevents metabolic diseases in mice fed a high-fat diet. *Cell metabolism*, 15(6), pp.848–860.

42 Burgoine, T., Forouhi, N.G., Griffin, S.J., Wareham, N.J. and Monsivais, P., 2014. Associations between exposure to takeaway food outlets, takeaway food consumption, and body weight in Cambridgeshire, UK: population based, cross sectional study. *BMJ*, 348, p.g1464.

43 Moss, M., 2013. *Salt, sugar, fat: How the food giants hooked us.* Random House.

44 Steptoe, A., Pollard, T.M. and Wardle, J., 1995. Development of a measure of the motives underlying the selection of food: the food choice questionnaire. *Appetite,* 25(3), pp.267–284.

45 Zurer, P., 1996. Chocolate may mimic marijuana in brain. *Chemical & engineering news,* 74(36), pp.31–32.

46 Rolls, E.T. and McCabe, C., 2007. Enhanced affective brain representations of chocolate in cravers vs. noncravers. *European Journal of Neuroscience,* 26(4), pp.1067–1076.

47 Bowen, D., Green, P., Vizenor, N., Vu, C., Kreuter, P. and Rolls, B., 2003. Effects of fat content on fat hedonics: cognition or taste?. *Physiology & behavior,* 78(2), pp.247–253.

48 Rozin, P., Ashmore, M. and Markwith, M., 1996. Lay American conceptions of nutrition: dose insensitivity, categorical thinking, contagion, and the monotonic mind. *Health Psychology,* 15(6), p.438–447.

49 Ramanathan, S. and Williams, P., 2007. Immediate and delayed emotional consequences of indulgence: The moderating influence of personality type on mixed emotions. *Journal of Consumer Research,* 34(2), pp.212–223.

50 Wilcox, K., Vallen, B., Block, L. and Fitzsimons, G.J., 2009. Vicarious goal fulfillment: When the mere presence of a healthy option leads to an ironically indulgent decision. *Journal of Consumer Research,* 36(3), pp.380–393.

51 Finkelstein, S.R. and Fishbach, A., 2010. When healthy food makes you hungry. *Journal of Consumer Research,* 37(3), pp.357–367.

52 Perloff, R.M., 2014. Social media effects on young women's body image concerns: Theoretical perspectives and an agenda for research. *Sex Roles,* 71(11–12), pp.363–377.

53 Barlett, C.P., Vowels, C.L. and Saucier, D.A., 2008. Meta-analyses of the effects of media images on men's body-image concerns. *Journal of Social and Clinical Psychology,* 27(3), pp.279–310.

54 Olivardia, R., Pope Jr, H.G., Borowiecki III, J.J. and Cohane, G.H., 2004. Biceps and Body Image: The Relationship Between Muscularity and Self-Esteem, Depression, and Eating Disorder Symptoms. *Psychology of men & masculinity,* 5(2), p.112.

55 McDool, E., Powell, P., Roberts, J. and Taylor, K., 2016. Social Media Use and Children's Wellbeing. *Sheffield Economics Research Paper Series.*

56 Spence, C., Okajima, K., Cheok, A.D., Petit, O. and Michel, C., 2016. Eating with our eyes: From visual hunger to digital satiation. *Brain and cognition,* 110, pp.53–63.

57 Pope, L., Latimer, L. and Wansink, B., 2015. Viewers vs. Doers. The relationship between watching food television and BMI. *Appetite,* 90, pp.131–135.

58 Franks, P.W. and Ling, C., 2010. Epigenetics and obesity: the devil is in the details. *BMC medicine,* 8(1), p.88.

59 Baumeister, R.F., Vohs, K.D. and Tice, D.M., 2007. The strength model of self-control. *Current directions in psychological science,* 16(6), pp.351–355.

60 Gailliot, M.T., Baumeister, R.F., DeWall, C.N., Maner, J.K., Plant, E.A., Tice, D.M., Brewer, L.E. and Schmeichel, B.J., 2007. Self-control relies on glucose as a limited energy source: willpower is more than a metaphor. *Journal of personality and social psychology*, *92*(2), p.325.

61 Wing, R.R. and Hill, J.O., 2001. Successful weight loss maintenance. *Annual review of nutrition*, *21*(1), pp.323–341.

62 Polivy, J. and Herman, C.P., 1999. The effects of resolving to diet on restrained and unrestrained eaters: the "false hope syndrome". *International Journal of Eating Disorders*, *26*(4), pp.434–447.

63 Burke, L.E., Wang, J. and Sevick, M.A., 2011. Self-monitoring in weight loss: a systematic review of the literature. *Journal of the American Dietetic Association*, *111*(1), pp.92–102.

64 Wing, R.R. and Phelan, S., 2005. Long-term weight loss maintenance. *The American journal of clinical nutrition*, *82*(1), pp.222S–225S.

65 Burke, L.E., Wang, J. and Sevick, M.A., 2011. Self-monitoring in weight loss: a systematic review of the literature. *Journal of the American Dietetic Association*, *111*(1), pp.92–102.

66 Parker, G., Parker, I. and Brotchie, H., 2006. Mood state effects of chocolate. *Journal of affective disorders*, *92*(2), pp.149–159.

67 Dallman, M.F., Pecoraro, N., Akana, S.F., La Fleur, S.E., Gomez, F., Houshyar, H., Bell, M.E., Bhatnagar, S., Laugero, K.D. and Manalo, S., 2003. Chronic stress and obesity: a new view of "comfort food". *Proceedings of the National Academy of Sciences*, *100*(20), pp.11696–11701.

68 Phillips, E.G., Wells, M.T., Winston, G., Ramos, R., Devine, C.M., Wethington, E., Peterson, J.C., Wansink, B. and Charlson, M., 2017. Innovative approaches to weight loss in a high-risk population: The small changes and lasting effects (SCALE) trial. *Obesity*, *25*(5), pp.833–841.

69 Piqueras-Fiszman, B., Alcaide, J., Roura, E. and Spence, C., 2012. Is it the plate or is it the food? Assessing the influence of the color (black or white) and shape of the plate on the perception of the food placed on it. *Food Quality and Preference*, *24*(1), pp.205–208.

70 Wansink, B. and Cheney, M.M., 2005. Super bowls: serving bowl size and food consumption. *Jama*, *293*(14), pp.1723–1728.

71 Wansink, B., Hanks, A.S. and Kaipainen, K., 2016. Slim by design: Kitchen counter correlates of obesity. *Health Education & Behavior*, *43*(5), pp.552–558.

72 Ogden, J., Coop, N., Cousins, C., Crump, R., Field, L., Hughes, S. and Woodger, N., 2013. Distraction, the desire to eat and food intake. Towards an expanded model of mindless eating. *Appetite*, *62*, pp.119–126.

73 Marie-Pierre St-Onge, Amy L Roberts, Jinya Chen, Michael Kelleman, Majella O'Keeffe, Arindam RoyChoudhury, and Peter JH Jones Short sleep duration increases

energy intakes but does not change energy expenditure in normal-weight individuals. *Am J Clin Nutr 2011 94* (2) 410–416 doi: 10.3945/ajcn.111.013904

74 Cunnington, D., Junge, M.F. and Fernando, A.T., 2013. Insomnia: prevalence, consequences and effective treatment. *The Medical Journal of Australia, 199*(8), pp.S36–40.

75 St-Onge, M.P., McReynolds, A., Trivedi, Z.B., Roberts, A.L., Sy, M. and Hirsch, J., 2012. Sleep restriction leads to increased activation of brain regions sensitive to food stimuli. *The American journal of clinical nutrition, 95*(4), pp.818–824.

76 Gonnissen, H.K., Hursel, R., Rutters, F., Martens, E.A. and Westerterp-Plantenga, M.S., 2013. Effects of sleep fragmentation on appetite and related hormone concentrations over 24 h in healthy men. *British Journal of Nutrition, 109*(4), pp.748–756.

77 Zheng, Y., Burke, L.E., Danford, C.A., Ewing, L.J., Terry, M.A. and Sereika, S.M., 2016. Patterns of self-weighing behavior and weight change in a weight loss trial. *International Journal of Obesity, 40*(9), pp.1392–1396.

78 Tal, A. and Wansink, B., 2013. Fattening fasting: hungry grocery shoppers buy more calories, not more food. *JAMA internal medicine, 173*(12), pp.1146–1148.

79 Wansink, B., Soman, D. and Herbst, K.C., 2017. Larger partitions lead to larger sales: Divided grocery carts alter purchase norms and increase sales. *Journal of Business Research, 75*, pp.202–209.

80 Wansink, B., Painter, J.E. and Lee, Y.K., 2006. The office candy dish: proximity's influence on estimated and actual consumption. *International journal of obesity, 30*(5), pp.871–875.

81 Levine, J., Baukol, P. and Pavlidis, I., 1999. The energy expended in chewing gum. *New England Journal of Medicine, 341*(27), pp.2100–2100.

82 Wansink, B., 2004. Environmental factors that increase the food intake and consumption volume of unknowing consumers. *Annu. Rev. Nutr., 24*, pp.455–479.

83 Wansink, B. and Shimizu, M., 2013. Eating Behaviors and the Number of Buffet Trips. *American journal of preventive medicine, 44*(4), pp.e49–e50.

84 Wansink, B. and Hanks, A.S., 2013. Slim by design: serving healthy foods first in buffet lines improves overall meal selection. *PloS one, 8*(10), p.e77055.

85 Swift, D.L., Johannsen, N.M., Lavie, C.J., Earnest, C.P. and Church, T.S., 2014. The role of exercise and physical activity in weight loss and maintenance. *Progress in cardiovascular diseases, 56*(4), pp.441–447.

86 Thomas, L.V., Ockhuizen, T. and Suzuki, K., 2014. Exploring the influence of the gut microbiota and probiotics on health: a symposium report. *British Journal of Nutrition, 112*(S1), pp.S1–S18.

87 Kratz, M., Baars, T. and Guyenet, S., 2013. The relationship between high-fat dairy consumption and obesity, cardiovascular, and metabolic disease. *European journal of nutrition, 52*(1), pp.1–24.

88 Eiler, W.J., Džemidžić M., Case, K.R., Soeurt, C.M., Armstrong, C.L., Mattes, R.D., O'Connor, S.J., Harezlak, J., Acton, A.J., Considine, R.V. and Kareken, D.A., 2015. The apéritif effect: Alcohol's effects on the brain's response to food aromas in women. *Obesity, 23*(7), pp.1386–1393.

89 Wildschut T, Sedikides C, Arndt J, Routledge C., 2006Nostalgia: content, triggers, functions. *Journal of personality and social psychology, 91*(5), 975

90 Legoff, D.B. and Sherman, M., 2006. Long-term outcome of social skills intervention based on interactive LEGO© play. *Autism, 10*(4), pp.317–329.

91 Brom, M., Both, S., Laan, E., Everaerd, W. and Spinhoven, P., 2014. The role of conditioning, learning and dopamine in sexual behavior: A narrative review of animal and human studies. *Neuroscience & Biobehavioral Reviews, 38*, pp.38–59.

92 Brody, S., 2010. The relative health benefits of different sexual activities. *The Journal of Sexual Medicine, 7*(4pt1), pp.1336–1361.

93 Carmichael, J., DeGraff, W.G., Gazdar, A.F., Minna, J.D. and Mitchell, J.B., 1987. Evaluation of a tetrazolium-based semiautomated colorimetric assay: assessment of chemosensitivity testing. *Cancer research, 47*(4), pp.936–942.

94 Amanda M. Brouwer, Katie E. Mosack., 2015 Motivating Healthy Diet Behaviors: The Self-as-Doer Identity. *Self and Identity, 14* (6): 638

95 Coughlin, S.S., Whitehead, M., Sheats, J.Q., Mastromonico, J., Hardy, D. and Smith, S.A., 2015. Smartphone applications for promoting healthy diet and nutrition: a literature review. *Jacobs journal of food and nutrition, 2*(3), p.021.

96 Chung, C.F., Agapie, E., Schroeder, J., Mishra, S., Fogarty, J. and Munson, S.A., 2017, May. When Personal Tracking Becomes Social: Examining the Use of Instagram for Healthy Eating. In *Proceedings of the 2017 CHI Conference on Human Factors in Computing Systems* (pp. 1674–1687). ACM.

97 Moro, T., Tinsley, G., Bianco, A., Marcolin, G., Pacelli, Q.F., Battaglia, G., Palma, A., Gentil, P., Neri, M. and Paoli, A., 2016. Effects of eight weeks of time-restricted feeding (16/8) on basal metabolism, maximal strength, body composition, inflammation, and cardiovascular risk factors in resistance-trained males. *Journal of translational medicine, 14*(1), p.290.

98 Wansink, B. and Van Ittersum, K., 2005. Shape of glass and amount of alcohol poured: comparative study of effect of practice and concentration. *BMJ, 331*(7531), pp.1512–1514.

99 Wansink, B. and Van Ittersum, K., 2003. Bottoms up! The influence of elongation on pouring and consumption volume. *Journal of consumer research, 30*(3), pp.455–463.

100 Whitfield, T.W. and Whiltshire, T.J., 1990. Color psychology: a critical review. *Genetic, social, and general psychology monographs. 116*(4), 385–411.

101 Koven, N.S. and Abry, A.W., 2015. The clinical basis of orthorexia nervosa: emerging perspectives. *Neuropsychiatric disease and treatment, 11*, p.385.

102 Carney, D.R., Cuddy, A.J. and Yap, A.J., 2010. Power posing: Brief nonverbal displays affect neuroendocrine levels and risk tolerance. *Psychological science, 21*(10), pp.1363–1368.

103 Mitchell, M.A. and Wartinger, D.D., 2016. Validation of a Functional Pyelocalyceal Renal Model for the Evaluation of Renal Calculi Passage While Riding a Roller Coaster. *J Am Osteopath Assoc, 116*(10), pp.647–652.

104 Polivy, J. and Herman, C.P., 1999. The effects of resolving to diet on restrained and unrestrained eaters: the "false hope syndrome". *International Journal of Eating Disorders, 26*(4), pp.434–447.

105 Briñol, P. and Petty, R.E., 2003. Overt head movements and persuasion: a self-validation analysis. *Journal of personality and social psychology, 84*(6), p.1123.

106 Butler, A.C., Chapman, J.E., Forman, E.M. and Beck, A.T., 2006. The empirical status of cognitive-behavioral therapy: a review of meta-analyses. Clinical psychology review, 26(1), pp.17–31.

107 Gollwitzer, P.M., Sheeran, P., Michalski, V. and Seifert, A.E., 2009. When intentions go public: Does social reality widen the intention-behavior gap?. *Psychological science, 20*(5), pp.612–618.

108 Turner-McGrievy, G.M. and Tate, D.F., 2013. Weight loss social support in 140 characters or less: use of an online social network in a remotely delivered weight loss intervention. *Translational behavioral medicine, 3*(3), pp.287–294.

109 Patel, S.R. and Hu, F.B., 2008. Short sleep duration and weight gain: a systematic review. *Obesity, 16*(3), pp.643–653.

110 Stapleton, P., Sheldon, T., Porter, B. and Whitty, J., 2011. A randomised clinical trial of a meridian-based intervention for food cravings with six-month follow-up. *Behaviour Change, 28*(1), pp.1–16.

111 Kraft, T.L. and Pressman, S.D., 2012. Grin and bear it: The influence of manipulated facial expression on the stress response. *Psychological science, 23*(11), pp.1372–1378.

112 Steptoe, A., Gibson, E.L., Vounonvirta, R., Williams, E.D., Hamer, M., Rycroft, J.A., Erusalimsky, J.D. and Wardle, J., 2007. The effects of tea on psychophysiological stress responsivity and post-stress recovery: a randomised double-blind trial. *Psychopharmacology, 190*(1), pp.81–89.

113 Sakulku, J. and Alexander, J., 2011. The impostor phenomenon. *International Journal of Behavioral Science (IJBS), 6*(1).

114 Gravois, J., 2007. You're Not Fooling Anyone. *Chronicle of Higher Education, 54*(11).

115 Smit, H.J., Kemsley, E.K., Tapp, H.S. and Henry, C.J.K., 2011. Does prolonged chewing reduce food intake? Fletcherism revisited. *Appetite, 57*(1), pp.295–298.

116 Patrick, V.M. and Hagtvedt, H., 2012. "I don't" versus "I can't": When empowered refusal motivates goal-directed behavior. *Journal of Consumer Research, 39*(2), pp.371–381.

117 Sharma, M., 2014. Yoga as an alternative and complementary approach for stress management: a systematic review. *Journal of Evidence-Based Complementary & Alternative Medicine*, 19(1), pp.59–67.

118 Pascoe, M.C. and Bauer, I.E., 2015. A systematic review of randomised control trials on the effects of yoga on stress measures and mood. *Journal of psychiatric research*, 68, pp.270–282.

119 Cohen, G.L. and Sherman, D.K., 2014. The psychology of change: Self-affirmation and social psychological intervention. *Annual review of psychology*, 65, pp.333–371.

120 Bellieni, C.V., 2017. Meaning and importance of weeping. *New Ideas in Psychology*, 47, pp.72–76.

121 Field, T., Hernandez-Reif, M., Diego, M., Schanberg, S. and Kuhn, C., 2005. Cortisol decreases and serotonin and dopamine increase following massage therapy. *International Journal of Neuroscience*, 115(10), pp.1397–1413.

122 Field, T., 2016. Massage therapy research review. *Complementary therapies in clinical practice*, 24, pp.19–31.

123 Campbell, R.S. and Pennebaker, J.W., 2003. The secret life of pronouns: Flexibility in writing style and physical health. *Psychological science*, 14(1), pp.60–65.

124 Lambert, G.W., Reid, C., Kaye, D., Jennings, G.L. and Esler, M.D., 2002. Effect of sunlight and season on serotonin turnover in the brain. *The Lancet*, 360(9348), pp.1840–1842.

125 Avery, D.H., Kouri, M.E., Monaghan, K., Bolte, M.A., Hellekson, C. and Eder, D., 2002. Is dawn simulation effective in ameliorating the difficulty awakening in seasonal affective disorder associated with hypersomnia?. *Journal of affective disorders*, 69(1), pp.231–236.

126 Hallam, R., Rachman, S. and Falkowski, W., 1972. Subjective, attitudinal and physiological effects of electrical aversion therapy. *Behaviour Research and Therapy*, 10(1), pp.1–13.

127 Wise, P.M., Nattress, L., Flammer, L.J. and Beauchamp, G.K., 2015. Reduced dietary intake of simple sugars alters perceived sweet taste intensity but not perceived pleasantness. *The American journal of clinical nutrition*, 103(1), pp.50–60.

128 Poncela-Casasnovas, J., Spring, B., McClary, D., Moller, A.C., Mukogo, R., Pellegrini, C.A., Coons, M.J., Davidson, M., Mukherjee, S. and Amaral, L.A.N., 2015. Social embeddedness in an online weight management programme is linked to greater weight loss. *Journal of The Royal Society Interface*, 12(104), p.20140686.

129 Hopkins, L.B., Medina, J.L., Baird, S.O., Rosenfield, D., Powers, M.B. and Smits, J.A., 2016. Heated hatha yoga to target cortisol reactivity to stress and affective eating in women at risk for obesity-related illnesses: A randomized controlled trial. *Journal of consulting and clinical psychology*, 84(6), p.558.

130 Genschow, O., Reutner, L. and Wänke, M., 2012. The color red reduces snack food and soft drink intake. *Appetite*, 58(2), pp.699–702.

131 Cho, S., Han, A., Taylor, M.H., Huck, A.C., Mishler, A.M., Mattal, K.L., Barker, C.A. and Seo, H.S., 2015. Blue lighting decreases the amount of food consumed in men, but not in women. Appetite, 85, pp.111–117.

132 Harris, M.A., Brett, C.E., Johnson, W. and Deary, I.J., 2016. Personality stability from age 14 to age 77 years. Psychology and aging, 31(8), p.862.

133 Roberts, B. W., Luo, J., Briley, D. A., Chow, P. I., Su, R., & Hill, P. L. 2017. A systematic review of personality trait change through intervention. Psychological Bulletin, 143(2), 117–141. http://dx.doi.org/10.1037/bul0000088

134 Schleider, J. and Weisz, J. 2017. A single-session growth mindset intervention for adolescent anxiety and depression: 9-month outcomes of a randomized trial. J Child Psychol Psychiatr. doi:10.1111/jcpp.12811

Acknowledgments

Our thanks go out to PR-supremo Mars Webb-Jones who played cupid at our first introduction because she had a hunch we would work well together. She was absolutely right. And to our agent, Antony Topping, for understanding and believing that Shrinkology would be so much more than 'just another diet book' and sharing our passion right from the start. But also to our husbands, Rik Mehta and Jonathan Woods, for their unswerving enthusiasm for this project and for happily keeping the home fires burning while we immersed ourselves in the Shrinkology world.